Praise for *The L*

"In this important book, David Agus—one of the most inspiring, practical, and knowledgeable people I know—shows us how to participate in the world of personalized medicine. It's easier than you think, if you have this book to guide you."

—Howard Stern, host of *The Howard Stern Show*

"Dr. Agus has done it again. *The Lucky Years* gives us a smart, informed, and sensible look at the latest medical breakthroughs and new technologies. Important and courageous, it tackles tough questions while showing us how to prolong the quality and length of our lives."

—Walter Isaacson, author of *Steve Jobs*
and *The Innovators*

"We all have a vague sense that there is a revolution underway in the world of biology and medicine. We hear about major innovations like the sequencing of the genome, targeted drugs, and big data. But what to make of them? How will they improve our health and change our lives? We could not have a better guide to make sense of it all than David Agus. In this fascinating and illuminating book, David brings together a deep knowledge of science, good writing, and common sense. We are lucky to have him around."

—Fareed Zakaria, host of *Fareed Zakaria GPS*

"*The Lucky Years* is an important and courageous book, raising big questions about health, longevity, and what it means to live a meaningful life. With a reverence for data and the latest science, Dr. Agus gives us his vision for a bright future of health, helping everybody understand how to navigate their options in the way that's best for them—and their loved ones."

—Arianna Huffington, editor-in-chief of
The Huffington Post and author of *Thrive*

"Dr. Agus offers an optimistic exploration of the new opportunities becoming available to us as exciting new technologies disrupt and revolutionize our understanding and practice of health care. Encouraging, but also clear-eyed and cautionary, *The Lucky Years* inspires us to take hold of the future of our own health—and, in turn, that of the planet."

> —Al Gore, 45th Vice President of the United States,
> Nobel Laureate in Peace, 2007

"Dr. Agus describes how a series of scientific breakthroughs enables everyone to lengthen and improve their lives—a future in which our body's natural mechanisms can be enlisted to fight disease and our genes can be edited to eliminate inherited ones. It is an inspiring vision."

> —Larry Ellison, cofounder and executive chairman,
> Oracle Corporation

"*The Lucky Years* is a steady dose of actionable knowledge about the one thing relatable to everyone: life. It's the doctor-patient relationship we all want and deserve. Dr. Agus is a trusted voice in a field of uncertainty."

> —Ashton Kutcher

"It sometimes takes a genius to know the difference between what's good and bad for us amid all the noise in health circles. Thanks, David Agus, for being that genius."

> —Michael Dell, founder, chairman, and chief executive
> officer, Dell, Inc.

"*The Lucky Years* inspires you to live a more healthful and meaningful life and provides practical and hopeful guidance for the path ahead. Dr. Agus will show you what it truly means to enjoy the lucky years."

> —Dov Seidman, author of *How: Why How We Do
> Anything Means Everything*

"Dr. Agus presents a provocative, highly informative way of understanding revolutions in health and health care today that will change the quality of our lives."

—Murray Gell-Mann, PhD, Nobel Laureate in Physics, 1969, and distinguished fellow and cofounder of the Santa Fe Institute

"Dr. Agus once again gives us a clear path to better health. We are lucky to have such an incredible guide to such a critical subject."

—Marc Benioff, chairman and CEO, salesforce.com

"[Dr. Agus] takes a hard look at the latest medical findings to show simple tips to living longer."

—*New York Post*

"If you have made a new year's resolution to get healthier, you'll find a buddy in David B. Agus's new book, *The Lucky Years*."

—*The Boston Globe*

"What is strongest here is Agus's deft marshaling of research old and new, and his common-sense guidance on preventives such as sleep hygiene and the optimal level of exercise."

—*Nature*

"Agus insightfully discusses how recent technological trends have the ability to boost both the medical industry's ability to effectively treat patients and its public perception, something that has incrementally declined through the last decade. . . . Highly informative. . . . Practical health information fortified with exciting news from the forefront of modern medical technology."

—*Kirkus Reviews*

Also by David B. Agus, MD

The End of Illness
A Short Guide to a Long Life

The
LUCKY YEARS

How to Thrive in the
BRAVE NEW WORLD
of Health

David B. Agus, MD
with Kristin Loberg

SIMON & SCHUSTER PAPERBACKS
New York London Toronto Sydney New Delhi

NOTE TO READERS

This publication contains the opinions and ideas of its author. It is intended to provide helpful and informative materials on the subjects addressed in the publication. It is sold with the understanding that the author and publisher are not engaged in rendering medical, health, or any other kind of professional services in the book. The reader should consult his or her medical, health, or other competent professional before adopting any of the suggestions in this book or drawing inferences from it. The author and publisher specifically disclaim all responsibility for any liability, loss or risk, personal or otherwise, which is incurred as a consequence, directly or indirectly, of the use and application of any of the contents of this book.

Simon & Schuster Paperbacks
An Imprint of Simon & Schuster, Inc.
1230 Avenue of the Americas
New York, NY 10020

Copyright © 2016 by Dr. David B. Agus

First Simon & Schuster paperback edition January 2017

SIMON & SCHUSTER PAPERBACKS and colophon are registered trademarks of Simon & Schuster, Inc.

For information about special discounts for bulk purchases, please contact Simon & Schuster Special Sales at 1-866-506-1949 or business@simonandschuster.com.

The Simon & Schuster Speakers Bureau can bring authors to your live event. For more information or to book an event contact the Simon & Schuster Speakers Bureau at 1-866-248-3049 or visit our website at www.simonspeakers.com.

Manufactured in the United States of America

3 5 7 9 10 8 6 4

The Library of Congress has cataloged the hardcover edition as follows:

Names: Agus, David, 1965– author. | Loberg, Kristin, author.
Title: The lucky years : how to thrive in the brave new world of health / David B. Agus with Kristin Loberg.
Description: First Simon & Schuster hardcover edition. | New York : Simon & Schuster, 2016. | Includes index. Identifiers: LCCN 2015033676
Subjects: LCSH: Health—Popular works. | Medicine, Preventive—Popular works. | Self-care, Health—Popular works. | BISAC: HEALTH & FITNESS / Healthy Living. | MEDICAL / Clinical Medicine.
Classification: LCC RA776.5 .A39 2016 | DDC 613—dc23 LC record available at http://lccn.loc.gov/2015033676

ISBN 978-1-4767-1210-9
ISBN 978-1-4767-1211-6 (pbk)
ISBN 978-1-4767-1212-3 (ebook)

To my dear children, Sydney and Miles:

On May 25, 1961, President John Fitzgerald Kennedy proclaimed, "I believe that this nation should commit itself to achieving the goal, before this decade is out, of landing a man on the moon and returning him safely to the earth."

On July 20, 1969, Neil Armstrong with the *Apollo 11* crew fought to land the lunar module before it ran out of fuel. Armstrong eventually took that first step on the moon. The average age of the remarkable team at Mission Control in Houston was twenty-six years old. That means the scientists and engineers in Mission Control were just eighteen years old when Kennedy made his 1961 statement. These teenagers who listened to President Kennedy were the future space program. Similarly, you and your generation are our future in health and medicine. We need you and are depending on you so we can continue the Lucky Years.

And to my partner, best friend, and wife, Amy:

Your love and support inspire me daily. I am so excited and privileged to continue to enjoy the Lucky Years with you . . .

... *most men and women will grow up to love their servitude and will never dream of revolution.*

—Aldous Huxley, *Brave New World* (1932)

Contents

ix

List of Illustrations

Page 72: Photo of Sir William Osler. Medical archives of the Johns Hopkins Hospital. Used with permission.

Page 73: Caricature of Sir William Osler. Medical archives of the Johns Hopkins Hospital. Used with permission.

Page 74: My Osler residency team. Medical archives of the Johns Hopkins Hospital. Used with permission.

Page 96–100: Examples of the Bills of Mortality. Courtesy of Jay Walker, the Walker Library of the History of Human Imagination. Used with permission.

Page 106: The illustration of the mitochondria comes from Wikipedia, https://en .wikipedia.org/wiki/File:Mitochondrion_structure.svg.

Page 110: The illustration of new reproductive techniques is an adaptation of a similar illustration featured in the article. Courtesy of author.

Page 126: Chart of life expectancy. Figures based on data from the Organization for Economic Co-operation and Development. Adapted from the *Wall Street Journal*, March 17, 2015. Courtesy of author.

Pages 130–132: Charts and Figures from the Task Force Report on Noncommunicable Diseases, copyright 2015 by the Council on Foreign Relations. Reprinted with permission. The data source is Institute for Health Metrics and Evaluation, Global Burden of Disease Study 2013.

Page 161: Cartoon of Jenner's inoculations. Public Domain. Wikipedia, http://en .wikipedia.org/wiki/File:The_cow_pock.jpg.

Page 189: Physical activity and life expectancy. Data from S. C. Moore et al., "Leisure Time Physical Activity of Moderate to Vigorous Intensity and Mortality: A Large Pooled Cohort Analysis," *PLOS Medicine* 9, no. 11 (2012): E1001335. Graphic courtesy of author and based on similar graphic in paper. National Cancer Institute and the Public Library of Sciences. Used with permission.

Page 191: Courtesy of Duke Medicine. Originally published in M. W. Dewhirst, et al., "Modulation of Murine Breast Tumor Vascularity, Hypoxia and Chemotherapeutic Response by Exercise," *JNCI Journal of the National Cancer Institute* 107, no. 5 (2015): djv040 DOI: 10.1093/jnci/djv040.

Page 203: Illustration by Habib M'henni, via Wikimedia Commons, https:// upload.wikimedia.org/wikipedia/commons/6/69/Obstruction_ventilation _apn%C3%A9e_sommeil.svg.

Page 226: Photo of the Kouros by Dorli Burge, via Wikimedia Commons, https:// upload.wikimedia.org/wikipedia/commons/c/c3/Kouros_Real_or_Fake .jpg.

Page 230: Photo of me courtesy of Sydney Agus.

The
LUCKY YEARS

Destiny of the Species

Welcome to the Lucky Years

O wonder!
How many goodly creatures are there here!
How beauteous mankind is! O brave new world,
That has such people in 't.

—William Shakespeare, *The Tempest*, act V, scene I

M iss Wanda Ruth Lunsford, twenty-six, must have been thinking about her own mortality the day she reported on a stunning experiment.[1] Picture two rats, one old and gray, the other young and vivacious. Now imagine joining them surgically at their sides by peeling away a thin layer of skin and neatly stitching the exposed surfaces together. Through this Siamese-twin-like junction, the rodents are able to share their circulation, pumping each other's blood and exchanging bodily fluids. Miss Lunsford and her colleagues wanted to see what would happen. Among the rats that survived the unnatural union, the geriatric ones physically turned into their younger counterparts, as if they'd tapped the fountain of youth. The elder rats gained shinier, more colorful fur and clearer eyes, taking on the general appearance of the younger rats hitched to their sides. A four-hundred-day-old rat, more or less akin to a middle-aged man, lived nearly as long as the spry counterpart to which he was attached.

When Miss Lunsford, a nutritionist and graduate student at Cornell University working in the lab of biochemist and gerontologist Clive McCay, shared these results at a gathering to focus on the problems of aging led by the New York Academy of Medicine, no one—not even Lunsford and her teammates—could explain this "age-reversal" transformation. The year was 1955, the same year the Food and Drug Administration approved the polio vaccine, the power of the placebo effect was first written about, Albert Einstein died at the age of seventy-six, and Steve Jobs and Bill Gates were born.[2]

Miss Lunsford's procedure, anatomically linking two organisms, had a name by then—parabiosis. But while this wasn't the first time it had been performed, her explorations were among the first to use parabiosis to study aging. And they weren't without their challenges. According to one description of the research, "If two rats are not adjusted to each other, one will chew the head of the other until it is destroyed."[3] Of the sixty-nine pairs of rats that Lunsford had helped conjoin in Clive McCay's lab, eleven died from a peculiar condition that developed about one to two weeks after partners were united; it was likely a form of tissue rejection. But the pairs that survived gave a glimmer of hope for reversing the maladies we all face.

In February of 1956, McCay, Lunsford, and a third Cornell researcher, Frank Pope, published their findings on the procedure's overall restorative effects in the *Bulletin of the New York Academy of Medicine* with an apt title: "Experimental Prolongation of the Life Span." In 1960, the results of Miss Lunsford's investigations in McCay's lab culminated in her thesis dissertation.[4] But the research didn't take off as you might expect in light of such intriguing findings. It pretty much sputtered and stalled for the next sixty-odd years. Interestingly enough, you can get a sense of the climate in which these scientists were working by reading a line in the opening paragraph of their paper: "Thus far man has made little progress in [studying aging] because human beings have chosen to expend their energies in improving the supposed comforts of living and methods of warfare."

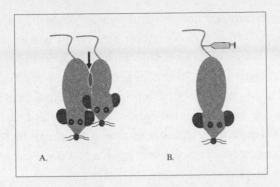

The studies done in laboratory mice indicate that young blood can reverse some signs of aging when given to an older mouse, suggesting that young blood contains "rejuvenation" factors. This figure demonstrates the two ways to reverse aging in the studies. (A) *Heterochronic parabiosis* is the process by which an old and a young mouse are joined surgically at the skin (where the arrow is pointing), thereby allowing their blood supplies to mix as the skin grows together. (B) Plasma from a young mouse (containing all of the proteins) is regularly injected into the tail vein of an old mouse.

When researchers at the University of California, Irvine, and the University of California, San Francisco, studied the life spans of old-young rat duos in 1972, they noticed that the older rodents lived four to five months longer than controls did.[5] This was another important clue suggesting that young blood might affect longevity if it's allowed to circulate in an aged animal. But that wasn't enough to stimulate the research in this area either, and parabiosis became obsolete. However, early in the twenty-first century, a Stanford stem-cell biologist brought the technique back to life. He was then working under a mentor who'd learned how to join mice together as a teenager in, believe it or not, 1955, while assisting a hospital pathologist in Montana. This ultimately paved the way for breakthroughs in cancer biology, endocrinology, and immunology today.[6, 7]

In 2014, researchers at UC San Francisco, Stanford, and Harvard each independently repeated Lunsford's nifty little experiment and discovered that you can reverse aging in older mice by hooking them up to younger ones and splicing their bloodstreams together.[8, 9, 10, 11]

So what is actually going on physiologically when the old and young combine? This procedure activates dormant stem cells in the older mouse, which turns back the clock and allows the stem cells to restore function to tissues. Stem cells are mother cells with the potential to become any type of cell in the body—from those that allow your heart to beat to brain cells that make you smart—and that also have the power to renew themselves or multiply. The surprising conclusion drawn from this recent parabiotic research is that the secret to reversing aging organs is lying asleep inside each of us!

Future research will figure out how exactly this age-reversal phenomenon works. In almost every tissue examined, including those of the heart, brain, and muscles, the blood of juvenile mice seems to "zap" new life into aging organs by awakening the sleeping stem cells through infusing substances normally associated with youth—proteins and growth factors that are particularly prominent in young blood but not old. Youthful blood sparks the birth of new cells in the brain and the system that governs our sense of smell. It's also been shown to reverse thickening of the heart's walls due to aging, increase muscle strength and stamina, and reverse DNA damage inside muscle stem cells. Young blood can promote the repair of damaged spinal cords in older mice and improve learning and memory. A study from a laboratory in Canada in 2015 reported that fractured shin bones of old mice healed faster and better when they were joined to young mice rather than to mice their own age.[12]

No one paid attention to Miss Lunsford's work in her day, with its air of science fiction, but everyone in the scientific world today is taking notice, and a groundswell of exciting new research is emerging. What was once an implausible, preposterous idea swiftly cast aside has become a hypothesis in need of serious validation. Are we "de-aging" animals? Are we resetting the aging clock? Or are we merely restoring function to tissues and helping them repair damage?

Human trials are now underway using plasma transfusions. Plasma is a clear straw-colored liquid component of blood that contains a complex mixture of substances and proteins, some of which help the blood to clot. Plasma is the single largest component of blood, but it's missing from traditional blood transfusions, in which only the red blood cells are transfused. For this reason, blood transfusions aren't fountains of youth. In 2015, a clinical trial in California became the first to start testing the benefits of young plasma in older people with dementia. Clinical trials in other disease areas are scheduled to begin in 2016. I am planning clinical trials in patients with advanced cancer that have failed treatments. Almost 90 percent of pediatric cancer is curable. If I can convince the body it is young again, maybe I can cure cancer.

Of course, certain problems still need to be worked out to prevent unwanted potential side effects, such as the body's rejection of the transfusion with a dangerous immune reaction. We also need to figure out how much and how often to give the plasma. Plasma from donors is also not a long-term or scalable treatment option. We first need to identify the active proteins and make them into drugs so they can be made available for large numbers of people. This will be a good thing, though, because it will prevent the development of a black market for plasma, whereby young and healthy children and teenagers bleed for the highest price. Or worse, supplies of fake or tainted plasma enter the market. These fears are not unfounded. Health is one of the most lucrative sectors for con artists and criminals.

And the fact that such therapies activate stem cells is also a double-edged sword. On the one hand, it gives an old body access to new and vibrant cells. But it also means that over a long period, cell division could run amok, and this has the potential to produce cancer and other disorders. Despite all this, the concept is promising on so many levels once we know how to minimize the side effects and potential for evil business trades, as well as maximize the benefits. So picture yourself receiving a dose of synthesized young blood or protein someday in midlife and in your golden years to stave off the Alzheimer's disease that runs in your family, to help you maintain your mobility, to speed up your metabolism so you can effortlessly lose and maintain your weight, to quash chronic conditions such as insulin resistance and diabetes, to clean your liver and arteries, to wipe out arthritis and revitalize joints, to balance your body's flow of hormones and its circadian rhythms so that you feel good all day long, to abolish gray hairs and return your hair to its natural color, to lift your spirits and stamp out your chronically bad mood, and to trigger your body to behave—and look—as if you are decades younger. This may be possible sooner than you think.

Welcome to the Lucky Years

We are indeed living in a *brave new world*, but this one won't be dystopian as the one Aldous Huxley portrayed in his famous book.

Chances are you stand to live a much longer, more enjoyable life than you ever thought possible—thanks not only to such age-reversing remedies as plasma transfusions, but also to a staggering volume of other new knowledge and technologies in medicine. Scientists are developing drugs to reverse once-fatal ailments such as heart disease and figuring out how to harness a person's immune system to melt away cancer. They are designing computer applications to help us regularly and effortlessly track key features of our biological functions including blood sugar, sleep quality, heart rate, blood pressure, stress levels, mileage, moods, and even risk for problems ranging from depression to cancer.

For the first time, we have at our disposal all the information we need to design our own health—and, in turn, the health of the planet. Put simply, people living in the twenty-first century are the most fortunate of all previous generations. That's why these are the Lucky Years.

If you are fifteen years old or younger and living in a high-income country, your chances of developing and dying from breast cancer, heart disease, lung cancer, or leukemia before your sixtieth birthday are declining dramatically. Despite much higher rates of obesity and physical inactivity, premature death and disability from noncommunicable diseases (e.g., heart attacks, chronic respiratory diseases, and diabetes) have declined significantly in the United States and other high-income countries, thanks to inexpensive and effective prevention, early detection, management, and treatment tools and policies. But more needs to be done, and it will come from us if we can do three things: believe that aging is optional, think about our future, and act on it today.

A Brave New Reality

The Lucky Years have been the destiny of our species for millennia. But there's a catch to benefiting from this new era. You as an individual and we as a society stand at a historic crossroads. Only those who learn how to think, act, and behave certain ways will reap the benefits of the tremendous opportunities afforded to us through the power of these medical revolutions.

Andy Grove, the former CEO of Intel and a pivotal early mentor of mine, once referred to an inflection point in the development of technology—a critical moment when the curve of progress versus time changes, the things that used to work don't work anymore, and new, necessary technologies become available. Individuals (or companies) that adapt to the shift and use those emerging technologies are wildly successful, and those that don't adapt fail.

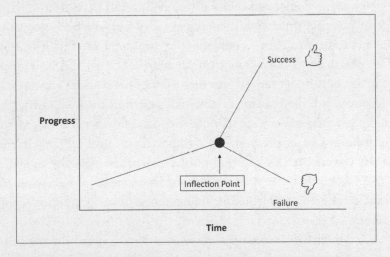

Andy Grove's concept of the inflection point in the curve of progress versus time, adapted from *Only the Paranoid Survive.*[13]

This concept is often used in business circles, but it applies to matters of health as well. The slope of the curve of progress versus time in medicine is changing rapidly, and we all must adjust our thinking and behavior to take advantage of what the Lucky Years offer to fight against disease and premature death. Hence, *The Lucky Years* is about this inflection point that is happening in health—and how to respond appropriately to the ongoing revolution. The costs of not doing so are too high.

Indeed, despite the spectacular volume of information on how to live better available in the past two decades, we continue to suffer from chronic, debilitating, and largely preventable conditions that strike us at increasingly younger ages. And as a cancer doctor who watches people die weekly, I think this is categorically unacceptable. I'm excited about the opportunities that we all have today. But I'm also worried that many people won't benefit from this medical revolution unless they have a certain knowledge base and the tools to take action. At the same time, we also need society to continually and speedily build the framework and allocate resources to enable further changes to occur. I hope this book will help us all do just that.

New technologies and constantly emerging data have produced the age of precision medicine, sometimes called personalized medicine. But precision medicine is still stuck in treatment mode—it's being used primarily to learn how to treat your condition precisely once you have it. It hasn't moved into the realm of prevention. However, it will, and it will shed the imperfections that distort the field today. For example, a major 2015 report published in the *New England Journal of Medicine*, one of the best, most respected medical journals in the world, warns that DNA testing results can be dramatically flawed.[14] These genetic analyses that profile your DNA are supposed to assess risk for numerous ailments including cancer, heart conditions, and Alzheimer's disease.

You'd think these screenings would be straightforward and unequivocal, as if you're reading a sentence that says, "You have a higher risk of breast cancer because you carry a defect on the BRCA gene." But when given the same test results, doctors interpret the data differently. Some say there's a higher risk or lower risk of developing a disease based on the same genetic defect. Unfortunately, not all gene mutations—variations in human DNA, or variants—are equal. *Mutation* carries a connotation of negativity and harmfulness, but that's not entirely accurate. Some mutations increase risk by a lot, while others barely nudge the risk meter or don't do anything. And most variants are unresolved—we don't know what they mean, which creates an even bigger dilemma for both doctors and patients. Complicating matters further, most variants are uncommon, so it becomes an even greater challenge to distinguish those that matter and determine by how much. Although the federal government helped create and finance ClinVar, a database for scientists around the world to collect anonymous gene findings, there's no federal oversight on the actual execution of the technology to push for better standards and a universal understanding of how one should interpret results accurately.

In fact, the use of many new medical technologies lacks proper oversight, and this can make them harder to put into effect or more prone to errors and misuse. In the case of DNA screening, companies are testing for lots of gene variants, many of which haven't been scientifically validated as to what they might mean in terms of risk factors for disease.

In the case of ClinVar, which became the basis for the review published in the *New England Journal of Medicine*, the project has documented more than 172,000 variants in nearly 23,000 genes.[15] This represents a mere fraction of the millions of variants known to exist, but at least they reflect some of the more common alterations. Nearly 120,000 of these variants can influence the risk for a disease. A few labs have analyzed a little more than 10 percent of these variants, allowing results to be compared. But they don't agree on what the variants mean in all cases. Some identified variants that raise risk while others said those very same variants had either no effect or an unknown effect. Different interpretations are currently found in more than 400 gene variants—interpretations that could inform a medical decision, such as whether to get a defibrillator implanted in your chest to slash the risk of sudden cardiac death, or to have healthy organs removed to lower the risk of certain cancers (e.g., breast and ovarian).

I've experienced the frustration of such fallibilities in my own family with a loved one who was tested for risk of Alzheimer's disease. The results of her genetic screening showed a higher-than-normal risk. She lived with the psychological weight of this outcome for two years until she was tested again, and another variant was then discovered that *protects* her from that devastating affliction.

On a similar note, I had a fifty-year-old patient with metastatic lung cancer—cancer that had started in his lungs and traveled to other organs in his body. The odds of survival in cases such as this are typically low. When I ordered a test to sequence his tumor from the hospital that had done his initial lung surgery, it was determined that there were no gene variants to target with drugs. But then I had another lab perform the testing, and the results revealed a variant to target. This man is still alive today, four years later, thanks to finding that target and using drugs that slowed the progression of the cancer. I'll be going into more detail about this kind of testing later in the book, as well as explaining more about what gene variants are and how they play into your fate. The point is, it's sometimes better to do no test than the wrong test, and you should never underestimate the value of a second opinion. In the future, however, such testing will become more absolute and reliable, lessening the need for second opinions.

It's Not a Right, It's a Responsibility

In the upcoming chapters, I'll also be presenting some of the bigger issues we have to understand and face in the Lucky Years. What are the ethical considerations of many of these advances? Should there be regulation? Who should lead these efforts?

Let me give you a prime example of losing in the Lucky Years amid great revolutions. Over the next decade, millions of people will achieve better health with breakthrough new medicines. But at the same time, millions more will also become victims of counterfeit drugs. Upwards of 40 percent of drugs in third world countries are fake, but even in the United States and Canada, doctors, pharmacies, and consumers have unknowingly purchased bad medicine due to weaknesses in the supply chain. It's easier to counterfeit a drug than money; all you need is a pill presser, available today online for less than $1,000. The stakes are high when you look at human lives, and particularly so in areas of medicine where people are desperate. How many patients in Boston and Baton Rouge have died from counterfeit drugs? One of our most important anticancer drugs, bevacizumab (Avastin), was counterfeited in 2011 and sold to Americans who ended up losing several months of their lives.[16]

We expend so much energy and brainpower to protect our bank accounts, credit cards, and other important things, yet we don't do the same for drugs. We also lack proper safety measures in the production and distribution of food, hence the routine headlines about tainted meat and dairy, expensive recalls, and scary salmonella or listeria outbreaks that kill vulnerable people, young and old. We need to bring technology into the food and drug realms or we are going to be in trouble.

We also need health care to be above politics. For example, consider newborn screening with heel sticks, a tiny sampling of blood drawn by pricking the heel with a needle, which started in the 1960s and became standard and mandatory across the country. Every child is screened now for more than thirty rare and life-threatening diseases. In the past, research has been done on those blood samples to provide information that's critical to improve the health of every child in this country. But in December of 2014, conservative lawmakers got their way when President Obama signed into law a bill requiring informed consent on every sample to be used for federally funded research. The new bill basically eliminated the research component to the blood draws because of the costs and difficulties involved with obtaining informed consent. Was anyone harmed by how the process worked for fifty years before that?

The answer is no, and thousands upon thousands of lives were saved with the information culled from those heel sticks, which not only alerted new parents as to their newborn's chances of having a genetic or metabolic disorder but also provided free, semi-anonymous data that fueled important research. (I say "semi" because individual names are redacted, but certain identifying features remain that are necessary for research, such as gender, age, and ethnicity.) One out of every 1,500 babies will develop a disorder detectable through newborn screening. Because most newborns tend to look normal, there is no way of knowing if a child has a problem until diagnosable, visible symptoms develop. By then, it may be too late to stop or reverse the effects.

Phenylketonuria, or PKU, is an example of one such inherited disorder that causes an amino acid called phenylalanine to build up in your blood. On soda cans you see labels warning people that the drinks contain phenylalanine, which individuals with PKU cannot metabolize properly. This is due to a defect in the gene that helps create the enzyme needed to break down the substance. If you don't know that your child carries the mutation for the disorder upon birth, then you won't know to avoid phenylalanine, commonly found in not just soda but many foods with protein. Serious developmental and intellectual challenges can result if a newborn with PKU isn't screened and identified quickly after birth.

We know a lot more about inherited disorders like PKU today, thanks to these universal screenings and the research they have fueled. But in 2015, a study of about 400,000 newborns in California could not move forward due to the impasse the new law created when more than half of the participants didn't sign the consent. So I ask: Do you want privacy above progress?

We allow people to drive their cars until they fail a portion of their test. If you're older and have a problem, you lose your license. Clearly, our behaviors affect other people around us when we drive. By the same token, our health affects other people. When we are sick and in need of medical care, it strains family members, society, and the government to some degree. We all pay.

We need to think of health care in the same way. Driving is not a right; driving is a responsibility. Likewise, health care is not a right; it's a responsibility. And step one in taking on that responsibility, both personally and for the sake of a healthier society, requires an important tool that this book helps you gain: an understanding of your personal context.

The Power of Context

When I have to tell patients and caregivers that I have nothing left to give them to treat a disease and that the end is surely near, I can't help but think: *What could I have done differently? What could they have done differently? What could have changed the course of their fate? Was there a clinical trial that could have helped them? How could they have delayed this unfortunate, agonizing premature death when they deserved more fulfilling years of life?*

And then I have to reconcile the fact that yes, there's a lot we all could have done, but the clear changes could have been in their lifestyle choices and even in their *thinking processes*. Here's what I mean by that: If you throw a lit match into a dewy wet forest, what happens? Nothing. But toss that same incendiary device into a parched landscape that hasn't seen rain in a long time, and you'll soon have a quickly moving fire on your hands. The difference between these two environments—one damp and saturated and another dry and thirsty—means everything in terms of how they respond to that spark.

I use this analogy frequently when I describe how one person can be diagnosed with cancer while another, perhaps even an identical twin, escapes such a condition. If I were to pluck at random one hundred people over the age of fifty from the streets of New York City and sequence their DNA, many of them will show mutations for genes that can trigger leukemia. But only a small fraction of them will ever develop it. What explains this? Again, go back to the image of the forest. One has an environment that effectively squelches the flame while the other has an environment that feeds it. In my world, in terms of the body, I call this "environment" *context*. Each one of us harbors a certain context we must honor in our health decisions. What's good for me might not be good for you, depending on each of our individual contexts. If we can know more about our personal contexts, we can make better decisions for ourselves.

An intriguing 2015 paper published in *Science* called attention to the fact that normal skin taken from people's eyelids—a common place for cancer-causing UV exposure from the sun—is already chock-full of potential drivers, or mutations, for cancer.[17] So while the gene alterations pointing to cancer are already there, these people didn't have skin cancers. Why not? Probably because the context wasn't right despite these mutations. UV radiation causes so many mutations that we would all have skin cancer all the time if there were an absolute and linear path between these mutations and the development of skin cancer. But that doesn't happen. Which points to the complexity of a disease like cancer and the complexity of its context—the human body. Quite simply, the DNA changes are necessary, but not sufficient for cancer to happen.

The concept of context cuts multiple ways. Your body today won't be the same in five, ten, and twenty years. Similarly, your body goes through different contextual phases during every hour of the twenty-four-hour circadian cycle. When you woke up this morning, various hormone levels in your body were totally different from where they are now and where they will be when you climb into bed tonight. At the same time, your DNA—your inherited code of life—is probably behaving differently right this moment than it will tomorrow, next month, or a few years from now. When I was in medical school, the prevailing wisdom said that DNA was, for the most part, fixed. But today we know otherwise. Just as information is fluid and dynamic, so is the readout from your DNA. What we eat, how often we get off our butts and break a sweat, what we're exposed to in our environment, how deeply we sleep, which drugs and supplements we take, and even the beliefs we keep in our minds all affect the expression of our genetic code. And this, too, plays into our context and risk for illness and disease.

Far too often, we are given one-size-fits-all health recommendations that don't necessarily consider our individual context. And indeed, there's a lot of noise out there in the arena of health advice. For every scientific article, for example, that tells the truth but remains buried in the literature, six others tell the untruth that the media likes to play up. For every person who says do this, not that, there's someone else saying exactly the opposite. And then at the same time we hear about impressive new technologies that might wipe out diseases like obesity and cancer. Question is, will they help *you*? Which research is actually promising and why? How does the average person access the most cutting-edge technologies and medicine? Which data-based medical ideas and applications are total bunk? What will our experience of a doctor's visit be like in the Lucky Years? And aside from high-tech strategies now or soon to be available, what low-tech habits should we all keep in the Lucky Years? You're about to find out.

The explosion of medical information has far outstripped our ability to process it. This is why we need a new way to make personal health choices. After all, we have already entered the Lucky Years, and those of us who have the information to take action will only get luckier. I can't reiterate this enough: your right to pass into the Lucky Years is not predicated on wealth, personal resources, or social status. In the old world of medicine, only those who could afford the surgery and expensive, exclusive therapies to look younger could benefit. But now the game has changed. The Lucky Years don't discriminate based on money. They're a privilege of the prepared and knowledgeable.

One of my goals is to show you why each person must consider participating in our great health care system for the benefit of all of us. After all, don't you want to be part of the cure to illnesses? You can be. My hope is that you can begin to experience life—and health—in a whole new light. In the words of Sir William Osler, the father of American medicine, "The value of experience is not in seeing much, but in seeing wisely." It's time for all of us to see ourselves—and the future of our health—wisely.

CHAPTER 1

The Century of Biology

The Cure Is Already Inside You

I'm fascinated by the idea that genetics is digital. A gene is a long sequence of coded letters, like computer information. Modern biology is becoming very much a branch of information technology.

—Richard Dawkins, British biologist and writer

Hardly a day goes by that I don't get at least one question about whether or not X, Y, or Z is "healthful." And yet I encounter a lot of skeptics and naysayers who want to go to battle against compelling, irrefutable data. It's disheartening to hear that public trust in physicians has plummeted over the past several decades.[1] In 1966, almost 75 percent of Americans said they had great confidence in the leaders of the medical profession; by 2012, that percentage had dwindled to some 30 percent. Why is this happening, and what does it mean for our collective and individual health? In another study, Princeton researchers found that people tend to regard scientists as they do CEOs and lawyers: all three types of professionals are perceived as highly competent but cold. Their work earns respect but not trust.

A couple of researchers at the University of Chicago in 2014 conducted a study of more than 1,350 randomly chosen Americans who provided written responses to questions. Astonishingly, half of Americans believe one of the following:[2]

1. Companies knowingly dump large quantities of dangerous chemicals into our water supply.
2. A US spy agency infected African Americans with HIV (and some are now saying that viruses with high mortality rates such as Ebola have been used for sinister purposes such as population control).
3. The government tells parents to give vaccines to their children even though that could increase their risk of developing autism.
4. US health officials withhold information about natural cures for cancer so that pharmaceutical companies can continue to profit.
5. The government and health officials pretend they don't know that cell phones can cause cancer.
6. Genetically modified foods (GMOs) are a plot to shrink the global population by delivering foods that can be toxic to unsuspecting consumers.

To my chagrin, the greatest proportion of people in the study—more than one third—believed that corrupt practices occur routinely in my line of work. They subscribe to the idea that the FDA deliberately suppresses information about alternative cancer treatments that don't entail drugs and radiation. Do any of these theories have merit? None do. Unfortunately, many people don't know where to turn for unbiased, trustworthy information, so these dangerous mythologies persist. And merchants of doubt and fear will keep these ideas alive.

After the publication of *The End of Illness*, my first book, I went through a revealing experiment. My credibility and "persona" were put to the test when four focus groups categorized by age (two groups of twenty-one- to thirty-nine-year-olds and two groups of forty- to sixty-year-olds) were exposed to a series of clips of me on various television shows. Then they were each interviewed about their general impressions of health and reactions to my message. Mind you, these were people who were chosen because they actively gathered information on health and wellness, and none worked in a health care setting. I won points for coming across as warm, trustworthy, passionate, and knowledgeable, but it didn't end there. I learned that Americans, broadly speaking, are inherently mistrustful of "experts"; they presume everyone is in someone's financial pocket and worry doctors could push drugs for kickbacks rather than solely making decisions in the patient's best health interest.

I also learned, this one to my surprise, that Americans perceive vitamins and drugs differently. They are psychologically averse to taking drugs, but not to taking vitamins. Why? Because, according to accepted wisdom, pharmaceutical companies promote drugs for *their* financial interests whereas purveyors of vitamins are motivated by *your* health interests. Suffice it to say, I walked away from the experience having learned that it's more important to express human concern than to launch into a jargonistic lecture about medicine.

It can be hard to change people's fierce beliefs about health, and that may be because holding on to them is part of our preprogrammed survival instinct. But we're no longer residing in caves. Now that we live in an era of abundant information and data, we need to develop a new survival instinct that's deft at navigating through the rapidly changing flow of information, some of it good, some of it not so good. Consider supplements, including those touted by popular physicians in the media. Most people are surprised to learn that supplements are almost entirely unregulated, so you don't know what you're really getting when you buy them, and their side effects and potential consequences to you could be hidden or, worse, unknown.

It's Complicated but Promising

One of my most important pieces of advice to people who seek the secrets to living long and well, and deciphering the good from the bad information, is to honor your body as an exceedingly complex organism with its own unique nuances, patterns, preferences, and needs. And there is no "right" answer in health decisions. You have to make suitable decisions for you based on your personal values and unique health circumstances as your context evolves and changes throughout your life. As it turns out, we're finally at a time in medicine where we can start to customize prescriptions for people—both general lifestyle interventions and specific drug and dosage recommendations to prevent, treat, or head off a disease. It doesn't matter if you call it personalized or precision medicine. The goal is the same: to prolong the quality of individuals' lives by using their personal health profiles to guide decisions about the prevention, diagnosis, and treatment of disease. And by profile, I don't mean just one's genetic code.

More than a decade has passed since scientists sequenced the entire human genome of about 30,000 total genes and 3 billion letters, and since then we've made many discoveries about the power we can wield over our individual DNA. Disease cannot be predicted by genes alone, for our genes don't work in a vacuum. Instead, they are significantly influenced by complex interactions with our diet, behavior, stress, attitude, pharmaceuticals, and environment. Every day a new finding correlates these factors with risk for illness. So when a diagnosis does in fact come in, you probably cannot point the finger at any single culprit. The condition is likely caused by an elaborate network of forces interacting within the complex human body. And ultimately, the result is that certain genes get turned on or off, triggering pathways whose endpoints are illness.

Let's say you have a genetic vulnerability to stomach cancer and heart disease. Does this mean these ailments are your destiny? Far from it. Your lifestyle choices largely determine whether those inherited codes express themselves or not and become your liabilities in life. In other words, you get to choose—to some degree—how your DNA is manifested. Genetics account for about a quarter of aging—how fast or slow you age and whether or not you're still getting carded at age forty. Habits can sometimes trump genes when it comes to the pace of your aging and how long you live. The nature vs. nurture debate has been clarified by the science of epigenetics—the science of controlling genes through environmental forces, such as diet and exercise. But my thoughts on epigenetics aren't totally aligned with those of other doctors. I don't, for example, subscribe to the theory that doing X, Y, and Z can change gene A, B, and C to effect outcome D, E, F. This is a complicated area of medicine where the data is still elusive. That said, I do believe that none of us is necessarily a victim of our DNA. And a lot of the advice doled out amid the hand waving is often good general advice, such as "eat real food" and "move more throughout the day." Who can argue with that?

As an aside, I find it amusing that in the summer of 1960, at another meeting where Wanda Lunsford presented her reports about the power of parabiosis—which were largely ignored by the general media— findings from another rat study zipped out to the nation through the Associated Press.[3] To quote the news directly: "How to Live Longer? Slow Eating! An experiment on rats has yielded hope that overweight people can prolong their life expectancy by as much as 20 percent. The Secret: Eat half as much." Again, can we argue with that? So we can be the architects of our own future health, so long as we're realistic about what we can control or hope to control.

Now, sometimes certain genes are, in and of themselves, enough to cause disease regardless of how we live. But the vast majority of conditions commonly diagnosed today are those that result from the intricate play between genes and the body's contextualized environment. This helps explain why most of the women diagnosed with breast cancer, or any degenerative condition for that matter, don't carry any inherited genetic mutations associated with the disease, nor do they have a family history of it. For example, Angelina Jolie's double mastectomy in 2013 was the right choice for her because she had a genetic mutation known to dramatically increase the likelihood of breast (and ovarian) cancer, but this is uncommon; only 5 percent to 10 percent of breast cancer cases in women are attributed to a harmful mutation in BRCA1 and/or BRCA2 genes. Most women who have a mastectomy choose to do it for other reasons. And those who opt for a double mastectomy due to cancer in one breast but who don't carry faulty genes linked to breast cancer will only increase their chances of survival negligibly—less than 1 percent over twenty years.

Heart disease, for another example, remains our number one killer for both men and women, but the most common causes of heart disease are not congenital heart defects. They are factors such as smoking, excessive use of alcohol or drug abuse, and the downstream effects of poor diet and unremitting stress, obesity, diabetes, and high blood pressure. Note that these are all factors that change a person's context. In 2015, the number of obese individuals in the United States as measured by body mass index (BMI) finally overtook the number of people who are overweight. That wasn't the year that people's genes changed to code for obesity. Something in their environment—in their context—changed, leading to more obesity, which is defined as having a BMI of 30 or above. While that sounds like terrible news, the silver lining is that such variables as the environment are often *changeable*, thereby making the outcome—obesity—*reversible*. And that's the kind of positive thinking we need going forward. Alongside that positive thinking will be new technologies that make ending obesity, as well as other maladies, possible.

Do you need to have your DNA profiled today? Not necessarily. My whole point is to show you how to take advantage of the most accessible, inexpensive tools in understanding your health and your health care needs. Besides, in the future doctors won't have to analyze your entire genome. They'll be able to use a simple blood test to look for genetic markers that are associated with certain risk factors. We already know of about three hundred markers that matter to human health. And dozens more will soon follow, if they haven't already by the time you read this book.

I am confident that within five to ten years, each one of us can be living a life of prevention that's so attuned to our individual contexts that diseases of today will be virtually eradicated. But this requires that we each get started now.

Steve Jobs's Other Legacy

In 2007, I was asked to be on Steve Jobs's medical team to help with his care and serve as a sounding board for him to discuss all the specialists he had in his circle. He was trying to stay as many steps ahead of his cancer as possible. This particular cadre of specialists not only included a handful of doctors from Stanford, close to where Steve lived and worked, but also entailed collaborations with Johns Hopkins and the Broad Institute of MIT and Harvard, as well as the liver transplant program of the University of Tennessee. We took an aggressive, integrated approach that leveraged the best anticancer technology at our disposal. This meant sequencing his tumors' genes so we could pick specific drugs that would target the defects in the cells that made them rogue. It was a revolutionary approach and totally different from conventional therapy, which generally attacks cell division in all of a body's cells, striking healthy ones along with cancerous ones.

For us on his medical team, it was like playing chess. We'd make our move with a certain cocktail of drugs, some of which were novel and just in development, and then wait to see what the cancer would do next. When it mutated and found a crafty way to circumvent the impact of the drugs we were using, we'd find another combination to throw at the cancer in our next chess move. I'll never forget the day we doctors huddled in a hotel room with Steve to go over the results of the genetic sequencing for his cancer.

This type of sequencing isn't as black-and-white as you might think. Just as interpreting someone's genetic profile can be subjective, so can the actual sequencing. Even the best gene sequencers from different institutions can find slightly different DNA portraits for the same exact patient, which is what happened with Steve's screening. After Steve verbally criticized some of us for using Microsoft PowerPoint rather than Apple's Keynote for our presentations, he learned that Harvard's results from testing his tumor's DNA didn't line up exactly with those from Johns Hopkins. This made our strategizing all the more challenging and demanded that we all get together to go over the molecular data and agree on a game plan.

I wish we could have saved him or turned his cancer into a chronic condition that could be controlled at the molecular level so he could go on to live a longer life and eventually die of something else. I have faith that one day cancer will be a manageable condition much in the way people can live with arthritis or type 1 diabetes for a long time before succumbing to, say, an age-related heart attack or stroke. Imagine being able to edit not only your own genes to live longer, but those of a cancer to keep it at bay, silence its copying power, and stop it in its tracks. From a rudimentary perspective, genes are your body's instructions, encoded in DNA. And cancer involves genes with a defect or defects that enable the "bad" cells containing those genes to block their own death or to continually divide, creating more rogue cells that can then maim the body's tissues and functionality. So with molecular anticancer therapies, it'll be like fixing the typos and misspellings in your personal "document" to live as long as humanly possible. Cancer will become a manageable life sentence, not a death sentence.

One genetic editing tool already exists. It's called CRISPR, which stands for Clustered Regularly Interspaced Short Palindromic Repeats. This genome editing tool is remarkably easy to use and effective, but it raises many concerns because of its ability to alter human DNA in a way that can be passed along to one's children and future generations. On the one hand, it can be used to cure diseases inherited from birth or acquired in life. In a fantastic review of the technology for the *New England Journal of Medicine*, Dr. Eric Lander, director of MIT and Harvard's Broad Institute, describes some of its utility:

> Genome editing also holds great therapeutic promise. To treat human immunodeficiency virus (HIV) infection, physicians might edit a patient's immune cells to delete the *CCR5* gene, conferring the resistance to HIV carried by the 1 percent of the US population lacking functional copies of this gene. To treat

progressive blindness caused by dominant forms of retinitis pigmentosa, they might inactivate the mutant allele in retinal cells. . . . Editing of blood stem cells might cure sickle cell anemia and hemophilia.[4]

But where there's a yin, there's a yang. The other side of this story is that this incredibly powerful technology can be used to control qualities that were previously uncontrollable, such as intelligence, athleticism, and beauty. And we just don't know what revising the human genome to create permanent genetic modifications might mean for future generations. What if you edit one part of the gene to reduce the risk of X but then inadvertently increase the risk of Y? As Lander notes, "For example, the CCR5 mutations that protect against HIV also elevate the risk for West Nile virus, and multiple genes have variants with opposing effects on risk for type 1 diabetes and Crohn's disease." Indeed, our knowledge is incomplete, but we'll be learning more as we move forward and try to deal with these possibilities—and challenges—on technical, logistical, moral, and ethical levels. I concur with Lander's concluding statement: "It has been only about a decade since we first read the human genome. We should exercise great caution before we begin to rewrite it."

Over the past few years, thousands of laboratories around the world have begun to use CRISPR technology in their research. In April 2015, Chinese scientists reported that, for the first time, they had edited the genomes of *human embryos*.[5] Wow! This was all made possible by a single discovery in 2012 by Jennifer A. Doudna, a biochemist at the University of California, Berkeley, who changed this field virtually overnight. Discoveries like this are now happening all the time around the world, and we need to be ready. It used to take a long time for new scientific knowledge or technologies published in the medical literature to enter mainstream medicine and fellow research labs, let alone the average doctor's visit. While it's been estimated that seventeen years usually passes before research evidence becomes part of clinical practice, that lag time will diminish quickly in the Lucky Years.[6] You'll be able to benefit from the findings of a new study or from a new technology in a matter of hours or days, not years or decades. But we'll have to figure out what to do with technologies like CRISPR before we unleash those into a clinical setting.

Unlike Jobs's binary world of computer programming, my field was a source of agony for him because I had to reconcile the hazy line between the science and art of medicine. He couldn't understand why I couldn't "debug" him like an Apple engineer.

But I learned again over those four years how important it is to tune in to your body. Steve had an admirable ability to listen to *himself* and know what his body wanted and needed. Although some will argue that he may have made some unwise choices early on in his fight against cancer—rejecting potentially life-saving surgery and turning to acupuncture, diet, and dietary supplements—that's not the point. I'm a firm believer that each one of us should be able to make our own decisions when it comes to our health. No one can take away the fact Steve was always true to his wishes, values, and personal health decisions. That he may have lowered his chances of survival by taking an alternative route first is immaterial. It was part of his journey, and he wasn't doing anything unethical. Steve was instrumental in choosing his therapy and his way of life from beginning to end. For him it was about how his choices made him *feel*. And he remained very much in tune with himself up to his last breath, letting that intuition guide his every action. I wish for that kind of mentality in not only myself, but in all my patients, friends, and loved ones.

Steve once said to me: "Health sounds like something I'm supposed to eat, but it tastes really bad." He made sure I kept the word *health* out of the title of my first book. But I'm using it this time in the subtitle because health has a different context now. We live in an exciting time, a world that is increasingly affording us all the opportunity to thrive for as long as we choose.

Old Wine in a New Bottle

At the end of the eighteenth century, the British scholar Thomas Robert Malthus wrote a controversial set of six books in which he meticulously calculated the end of the world based on the expanding population. At the time, the world housed 800 million people (to put that into perspective, that's a little less than half the number of people who used Facebook in 2015). He predicted that once the world population hit 2 billion, there would be apocalyptic famine and war. The planet wouldn't be able to sustain that number of people given its finite resources and arable land. Although Malthus's computations were incredibly accurate, and many contemporary people would agree with one of Malthus's assertions—"The power of population is indefinitely greater than the power in the earth to produce subsistence for man"—take a look around you. Obviously, we failed to elicit his predicted outcome, dubbed the Malthusian catastrophe.

In 2011, we surpassed the 7-billion mark, and we are headed to a whopping 8 billion by 2030, maybe sooner. Malthus could not have foreseen the impact that technological innovation would have. It has allowed us to thrive for millennia, and will continue to do so, but only if we prioritize it like never before. Yes, we need to fix global warming, develop plans for water security, solve poverty and pollution, end world hunger, prevent chronic disease, and discover new energy sources—and we can accomplish all of this through innovation in the Lucky Years.

The notion that experiments performed generations ago, like those of Wanda Lunsford, are relevant today should inspire great optimism. I only wonder how many other long-lost studies are holding the key to effective remedies and cures to our modern afflictions. And I also sometimes wonder if we have all the drugs we'd ever need to treat our ailments, but we just don't know which ones to try on which diseases.

For another example of old ideas once considered crazy or unbelievable gaining a new life in twenty-first-century medicine, take the story of William B. Coley and his "Toxins."

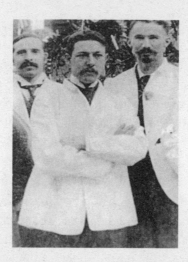

William Coley (center) in his surgeon's jacket attending a
Christmas party at the Hospital for the Ruptured and Crippled
(now known as Hospital for Special Surgery) in New York City,
1892.[7]

In 1891, while a surgeon at the New York Cancer Hospital (which
later became Memorial Sloan Kettering Cancer Center), Coley reviewed
the medical charts of patients with bone cancer and found the sarcoma
story of patient Fred Stein. Stein's cancer regressed after a high fever
from an *erysipelas* (now known as the bacteria *Streptococcus pyogenes*)
infection. The surgeon realized that this wasn't the first reported case
of cancer retreating after an *erysipelas* infection. Coley then deliberately
injected cancer patients who had inoperable, malignant tumors with live
bacteria first, then with dead bacteria. His thinking was that creating a
bacterial infection would stimulate the immune system, which in turn
would also attack the tumor. And it occasionally worked.[8] Some of
the patients' tumors vanished. For the next forty years, as head of the
hospital's Bone Tumor Service, Dr. Coley treated more than a thousand
people with cancers of the bone and soft tissue using his unorthodox
technique, dubbed immunotherapy—using the body's own immune
system to treat and sometimes cure a disease.

Coley's bacterial elixirs became known as Coley's Toxins, and they weren't without their detractors. Even though Coley and other doctors who used the toxins reported excellent results sometimes, Coley came under fire from colleagues who refused to believe them. The harsh criticism came at a time when radiation therapy and chemotherapy were developing, causing Coley's Toxins to disappear gradually until modern science could show that his principles were correct and that some cancers are sensitive to an amplified immune system. Today Coley is revered as one of the fathers of immunotherapy.

The field of immunotherapy has exploded in the last decade, especially as a method of treating fatal forms of advanced kidney cancer, skin cancer, lymphoma, certain lung cancers, and a few other cancers. Though more patients are benefiting, immunotherapy doesn't succeed in all cases. We need to learn much more if it will ever emerge as a safe, effective treatment for many different types of cancer. Currently, gains in survival can be seen in a patient where there are few to no effective treatment options and median overall survival is usually less than two years. In oncology-speak, *median survival* refers to the length of time from either the date of diagnosis or the start of treatment that half of the patients in a group of patients diagnosed with cancer are still alive.

Modern immunotherapy involves either infusing the body with a drug to unleash the body's own immune system to attack the cancer or injecting a special type of immune system cell called a T cell that has been taken from the patient and then modified in a lab to directly target and attack the cancer cells. These altered T cells become known as CAR T cells, short for "chimeric antigen receptors," which are proteins that allow the T cells to recognize and assault the specific protein on tumor cells, or antigen. These strategies share the same goal: harnessing the awesome power of the immune system to detect and attack cancer cells, which would otherwise flourish in the body undetected and unregulated.

The drugs getting the most attention are called checkpoint inhibitors. These release the natural brakes on the immune system so it can then launch an assault on the cancer. The treatment itself is called checkpoint blockage therapy. Two "switches" in the body, for example, that prevent tumor cells from attack by the immune system are labeled CTLA-4 and PD-L1. When these buttons are "on," the immune system is turned down so it can't recognize and kill cancerous cells. But when we disrupt these switches and block their functionality, this essentially enables the immune system's sentry—those T cells—to find and pummel the cancerous cells. It's important to note that cancer isn't a foreign mass of cells. It's our own cells run amok, hence it's difficult for the immune system to "see" them.

In one of the more extraordinary clinical trials taking place today, researchers at Duke University are using a different immune strategy by reengineering the polio virus. The idea of using viruses to attack cancer has been around for more than a hundred years, but we didn't have the technology or know-how to conduct these experiments until recently. The last case of naturally occurring polio infection occurred in the United States in 1979. These Duke researchers noticed something interesting about the virus: it kills cells by entering them through a "door" called a receptor. The special receptor for the polio virus turns out to be present on most solid tumor cells—lung, breast, brain, prostate—but not on most normal cells. The problem is that it can also attach to nervous system cells called neurons. When it kills them, the result is the muscular paralysis of polio. By extracting the disease-causing part of the virus that infects normal neurons, replacing it with the benign cold virus, and keeping only the part that attaches to and kills cancer cells, we can create a safe virus. Once injected directly into the tumor, it infects a few of the cancer cells and kills them while at the same time nudging the immune system. The immune system wakes up and thinks, *This is polio!* and kills the "bystander" tumor cells as well. The virus essentially tags the tumor as a "foreign" object and arouses the body's immune system to attack.

The studies using the polio virus have thus far been done mostly on patients battling advanced glioblastoma, one of the deadliest and most aggressive types of brain cancer, which often leads to death within weeks after standard treatments have failed. Researchers have managed to prolong the lives of some people by months, even years.[9]

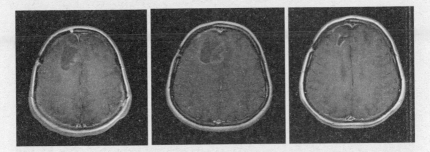

Brain scans of a twenty-year-old college student treated with the engineered polio virus (PVS-RIPO) by an infusion through a catheter directly placed into the tumor. The first panel shows the tumor (shaded area in upper left of the brain); the second panel shows the tumor after two months of treatment (where the tumor actually appears larger in size due to the inflammation of the antitumor response); and the third panel shows the tumor shrinking at nine months of treatment.

The idea that we can leverage our own immune systems to cure cancer is a romantic one, but it's not without its dangers. Our immune system, after all, is powerful on its own when allowed to operate at full speed. It can be risky to release its brakes, even in the hopes that it can clobber those devilish cells gone mad. Some patients who have tried immunotherapy died after developing devastating complications caused by an unrestrained immune system that indiscriminately attacks not only the cancer but also healthy and essential tissues and organs. Through ongoing clinical trials, researchers hope to overcome this challenge in the future. Immunotherapy is and will continue to be an important weapon against cancer, but it's currently limited in the cancers it targets and the patients it benefits. The challenge is to figure out in advance who will benefit. We also need to improve our understanding of which combination of checkpoint inhibitors or other immune-altering intervention best equips the body's immune system with anticancer ammunition.

As it happens, the more mutations a cancer has, the easier it often is to target with some immunotherapies because its cells become more "foreign looking" to the body's own immune system. Put another way, the more abnormal a tumor becomes, the harder evading detection by the immune system becomes, especially after some drug therapy puts that immune system on high alert and fits it with special "night-vision" goggles. This phenomenon was recently revealed in a standout paper for the *New England Journal of Medicine* by a team from Johns Hopkins Sidney Kimmel Comprehensive Cancer Center.[10]

DNA is constantly being repaired in the body, and the tools to do so are called "DNA mismatch repair." The Hopkins group looked at the presence or absence of DNA mismatch repair genes, which code for the system the body uses to recognize and fix bad DNA. They noted that regardless of the type of cancer, tumors that didn't have this repair system working properly were more likely to respond to the immune-brake system-altering, anti-PD-1 drug than those with tumors that had an intact mismatch repair. In other words, the worse the tumor cells were at repairing DNA, the better the patients responded to treatment. Immunotherapy likely won't stand on its own; it will be used in combination with other therapies, including chemo, radiation, and molecularly targeted drugs. But it will nonetheless become an indispensable tool made all the more powerful with adjunct weapons.

One of the surprising findings about immunotherapy is that many people who have tried it often report feeling better though their cancer is still there and may have even grown. But that's the problem with my specialty. Our only metric for success is shrinking a tumor. Slowing its growth, making somebody feel better, or watching a person continue to live longer than expected isn't classically accepted as "success" in cancer treatment.

If you come to see me in the office with a cancer that measures 5 centimeters, and if I give you a treatment, and when we remeasure the cancer in several months, it is 7 centimeters, did the treatment work? Would your cancer have been 15 centimeters without treatment? Most of the time with new drugs that stop or slow cancer, doctors and their patients are flying blind. In any randomized clinical trial, the drug might help a group of patients live longer, but it's very difficult to know what it's doing in the individual patient. Also, success will mean something different to each patient. If you can live another two good years, for example, on drug X, do you care how big your tumor is so long as you can tolerate the side effects and gain those extra quality years? I've never had a patient tell me, "I wish I had died last year." Even my sickest patients don't regret living longer than expected. They will do pretty much anything to live one more day, and they are often willing to try new strategies no matter how absurd they sound. They will, put simply, take risks with me in our fearless flight.

Good Bacteria Finally Gain a Good Reputation

Let's go back in time again. At roughly the same time Coley was experimenting with his toxins and trying to keep his critics from silencing his message, the Russian scientist Élie Metchnikoff was revealing how *Lactobacillus* bacteria could be related to health.

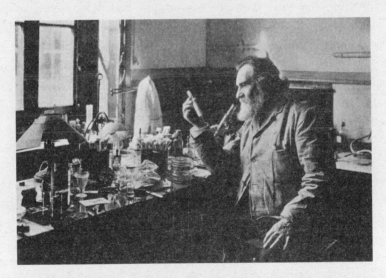

A photo of Élie Metchnikoff, father of natural immunity and 1908 Nobel Prize laureate in Physiology or Medicine, in his Ukraine laboratory.

Metchnikoff is considered the father of natural immunity. His work set the stage for the current popularity of consuming beneficial bacteria to nourish the gut's microbiome—the tribes of microbes in the intestinal tract that collaborate with your entire physiology. Metchnikoff predicted many aspects of current immune biology and was the first to suggest that we can benefit from lactic acid bacteria (or *Lactobacillus*). According to his theory, illnesses and aging are accelerated by the release of toxic substances in the gut by certain bacterial organisms, and lactic acid could prolong life by replacing the harmful microbes with useful ones. His ideas came from noticing the longevity of Bulgarian peasants and hypothesizing that it might be the result of their eating fermented milk products (principally yogurt). Metchnikoff himself drank sour milk every day based on his theory. More than a century ago, he said that "oral administration of cultures of fermentative bacteria would implant the beneficial bacteria in the intestinal tract." Yet only in the past decade has science validated and begun to understand Metchnikoff's bold assertions. In 2015, more studies emerged showing the power of the microbiome, some of which showed how certain foods you eat can change the composition of the bacteria colonies in your gut to either lead your body down the path to metabolic syndrome and obesity, or keep you slender and humming to the right metabolic tune.[11] We'll be exploring more about these findings and the microbiome in chapter 4. In the future, leveraging your microbiome for the better will likely be part of your health equation.

In 2008, the *European Journal of Immunology* paid tribute to Metchnikoff on the hundredth anniversary of his Nobel Prize in a beautifully written article chronicling his life and his contributions to society.[12] He was the first scientist to understand natural immunity to infection, the significance of inflammation, the role of digestion in immunity, the importance of gut flora, the implications of "self" versus "nonself" within the context of immunity so the body knows the difference between its own cells and foreign invaders. He even led the way in shaping the essence of the scientific study, for Metchnikoff taught how to go from observations to hypothesis for experimental testing. By the end of his life, he believed strongly in the power of ingesting good bacteria, principally *lactobacilli*, and he urged others to do so as well but was often ridiculed. Cartoons depicted him administering probiotics to people who wanted to live to one hundred.

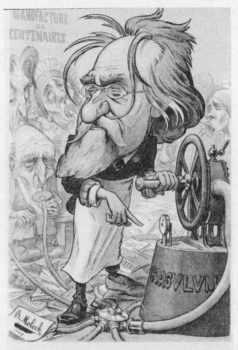

Le Professeur METCHNIKOFF

Metchnikoff believed his sour-milk (fermented) therapies could also help stop the aging process. When his
work in the area was described publicly, a French cartoon (shown here), titled "Manufacture de Centenaires,"
spoofed Metchnikoff's enthusiasm for probiotics as a
panacea, portraying him as one who would manufacture
centenarians.

If only he could see the world today! The scientific community is finally catching up with Metchnikoff's ideas. May other "old bottles of wine" from the past be uncorked to spill their wisdom in the Lucky Years.

Today, you might not know whether or not a glass of red wine at night is helping you, if a daily baby aspirin is a good or bad idea, or which probiotic could help your digestion. But sometime soon, a blood test will be all you need to find out what's best for you. Even without that definitive knowledge today, you can take action. While we await definitive studies demonstrating the impact of every aspect of your unique lifestyle and environment, we do have an enormous amount of evidence from other areas of medicine to help you make the best choices.

CHAPTER 2

This Isn't Science Fiction

The Power of Technology to Extend Your Life

It is much more important to know what sort of a patient has a disease than what sort of a disease a patient has.

—Sir William Osler

f I told you that you had to go to the doctor tomorrow to be closely examined and have a battery of tests—cholesterol, weight, blood sugar, liver and kidney function, metabolic health, cardiorespiratory fitness, blood count, cognitive function, perhaps even a DNA screening and check of your dental health—what would you do differently tonight besides brush your teeth for an extra minute? And what are you thinking about right now as you ponder this possibility? Are you nervous? Do you regret what you ate for breakfast or how you've lived your life this past year, maybe past several years? When you think about what you'll look like ten or twenty years from now and how your health will be, what comes to mind? If that's the hardest question to answer of all the ones I just gave you, you're not alone.

In 2013, a fascinating report was published in the journal *Science* by three researchers from Harvard and the University of Virginia.[1] One,

Daniel Gilbert, is a social psychologist well known for his research on such thought-provoking topics as what really makes us happy (not what you think), how we make decisions, and how well we predict what's called our "hedonic reactions" to future events. In other words, he examines the psychology of our future self: what we think our emotional state will be further down the road.

Now, if I asked you to give me a fair assessment of how much you've changed over the past decade, what would you say? My guess, based on Gilbert's results, is you'd admit to having changed a lot. But when asked about the next decade, you're more likely to say that you won't experience dramatic changes and that you've already become the person you want to be. That's what Gilbert discovered when he and his colleagues measured the preferences, personalities, and values of more than 19,000 people between the ages of eighteen and sixty-eight. He asked them two things: how much they thought they had changed in the past ten years and how much they thought they *would* change in the next ten. Surprisingly, it didn't matter how old his subjects were; the young, middle-aged, and older folks all believed they had changed a lot in the past but predicted that they wouldn't change much in the future. Apparently, we regard the present as a "watershed moment" at which we have finally become the person we want to be for the rest of our lives. And this natural tendency has many practical consequences. Gilbert writes:

> Time is a powerful force that transforms people's preferences, reshapes their values, and alters their personalities, and we suspect that people generally underestimate the magnitude of those changes. In other words, people may believe that who they are today is pretty much who they will be tomorrow, despite the fact that it isn't who they were yesterday.... [P]eople expect to change little in the future, despite knowing that they have changed a lot in the past, and ... this tendency bedevils their decision-making. We call this tendency to underestimate the magnitude of future change the "end of history illusion."

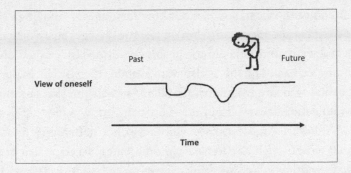

The end of history illusion states that the view of oneself shows no change going forward, and that one is only conscious of change in the past.

What I find interesting, and relevant to matters of health, is the following: "If people find it difficult to imagine the ways in which their traits, values, or preferences will change in the future, they may assume that such changes are unlikely. In short, people may confuse the difficulty of imagining personal change with the unlikelihood of change itself." [2]

Is this why it can be so hard for us to modify our behaviors to increase the chances of living longer and better? If seeing ourselves in the future is so difficult, then perhaps that's why it can be such a challenge and chore to make changes today. Try telling a rambunctious teenager to cut back on his sugar consumption, a twenty-something to curb the drinking at singles parties, an overweight forty-something to start exercising after twenty-five years of inactivity and a penchant for soda and fast food, or a sixty-something to give up the cigarettes she's smoked for four decades, and you can understand what I mean. The Gilbert research suggests that most of us believe we have attractive personalities, admirable values, and wise preferences. So given this state of affairs—having reached the "exalted state"—we might resist considering the possibility of change. We also like to believe that we know ourselves well, "and the possibility of future change may threaten that belief." Gilbert and his colleagues nail it perfectly when they write: "In sum, people are motivated to think well of themselves and to feel secure in that understanding, and the end of history illusion may help them accomplish these goals."

In the health realm, you can see how this kind of thinking can be a self-fulfilling prophecy: you don't make the changes that you should make and wind up reacting to the health conditions that await you as a result of your inaction. This is also what sustains the "It can't happen to me" mentality at any given time. We all make decisions that profoundly affect our future selves—from our daily habits to where we choose to live, what job we choose to have, whom we choose to marry, and even whether or not we choose to have children. But if we think that history is always ending today, then how can we make better decisions? How can we be motivated to make those necessary changes in our lives that make our futures better? According to Gilbert, we can blame the end of history illusion for our tendency to make decisions today that our future selves regret. I say, let's be more aware of this phenomenon and use it to choose wisely in the Lucky Years so we can maximize our quality of life later with no regrets. And one way I think we can do that is to understand and accept that we are all mightily complex systems.

You Are Complex and "Emerging"

Why we age is one of the most compelling questions we face. No one knows the answer or even how to define the process, but there are plenty of theories. Every day it seems a new study emerges to take a stab at what, how, and why we wear and tear over time to the point we can no longer replenish our cells, keep up with our biological housecleaning, and stave off degenerative illnesses. In a 2015 study, for example, research led by German scientists found that a certain area of the cell, the so-called endoplasmic reticulum, loses its powers in advanced age and this results in proteins not being able to mature properly.[3] At the same time, another area of the cell, the cytosol, accumulates the waste of oxidative damage. Although this interplay was previously unknown and now opens up a new understanding of aging, it doesn't tell the whole story. Nothing really will, because aging is not predicated on a single pathway.

Aging entails an opaque and exceedingly complex intertwining of different biological pathways. And the biological processes that underpin the illnesses of aging, from heart disease to cancer, vary enormously. However, the greatest driver of all—despite the wide spectrum of diseases and their inherent, unique mechanisms—is aging itself. Or, I should say, *old age*.

We do know that certain switches in the body turn on or off to effect changes that result in aging, especially once we've reached reproductive maturity in adulthood. In a recent discovery, scientists from Northwestern University found that a single genetic switch that exists in all animals, humans included, gets activated at some point after sexual maturity that essentially turns off a cell stress response that protects vital proteins.[4] Now if we can figure out how to turn this switch back on and protect our aging cells by boosting their ability to resist stress, we can keep our cells' quality control systems optimal and acting young.

We also know that changes to DNA—mutations—can lead to diseases such as dementia and cancer. Part of the programming that directs aging and dying lies in our genes, so we have to start looking at modulating genes—turning off the "die" or "age" switches—to extend life and increase not just the life span, but also the length of a healthy life. In worms, scientists can tweak certain genes and push the immortality button a little while longer. Why can't we learn to do that in humans?

While we tend to think of aging as a universal process of becoming increasingly less fertile, weaker, and vulnerable to illness, that's actually a gross misunderstanding, at least when you consider the aging process in species other than our own. It turns out that the phenomenon of aging shows an astounding diversity of strange patterns. This was recently demonstrated in a compelling 2014 paper written by researchers from a consortium of institutions including the University of Southern Denmark; the Max Planck Institute for Demographic Research in Rostock, Germany; the University of Queensland in Australia; and the University of Amsterdam in Holland, and published in the prestigious scientific journal *Nature*.[5] The authors describe how they studied aging in species ranging from lions, killer whales, baboons, lice, lizards, and nematodes to seaweed, oak trees, water fleas, frogs, and hermit crabs. The species included eleven mammals, twelve other vertebrates, ten invertebrates, twelve plants, and one algae.

For several species, the scientists documented what you'd expect to see with age: an increased risk of death, or mortality. In fact, most mammals, including killer whales and humans, as well as some invertebrates including water fleas, follow this pattern. But get this: some species' mortality *decreases* as they age. In other words, their chance of dying *declines with age.* And in some wild instances, mortality drops to virtually (and, obviously, theoretically) zero all the way up to death! Just who on this planet can do that? For desert tortoises and many plant species, both of which experience the highest mortality as juveniles, their mortality steadily dwindles as they age.

Amazingly, there are also species whose mortality remains relatively constant and unaffected by the aging process. They grow neither weaker nor stronger over time. This is most striking in the small freshwater animal *Hydra magnipapillata*, which has continuously low mortality. This creature can in fact be housed in lab conditions that render it effectively immortal. Some experts have calculated that 5 percent of the hydra population could still be alive after fourteen hundred years if they are kept in a certain environment that doesn't age them in a normal sense of the word. I know, this sounds like science fiction. But so did the thought of reversing aging in mice by hooking them up to younger comrades.

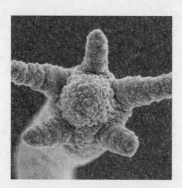

Scanning electron micrograph of the mouth and five tentacles of a freshwater *Hydra magnipapillata*. This species can practically live forever, at least relative to us.

Several species of plants and animals exhibit remarkably little change in mortality throughout their life spans. Examples include the plants rhododendrons, viburnums, and armed saltbushes; animals such as the hermit crab, common lizard, and red-legged frog; sea-dwelling life-forms oarweed (a type of kelp), red abalone, and the coral red gorgonian; and a few birds with some curious-sounding names such as the great tit and collared flycatcher.

If we were to look at the fertility patterns of the forty-six species these researchers studied, we'd find some surprising divergences from common beliefs about aging. Our fertility is high during a relatively short period of life, flanked by long periods of infertility before and after that window of time. The same pattern also occurs in other mammals such as killer whales, chimpanzees, and chamois, a goat-antelope species native to mountains in Europe, and in birds such as sparrow hawks. But some species actually become *more* fertile with age. Such a phenomenon is especially common in plants like the agave and in rare mountain plants. On the contrary, the nematode worm *Caenorhabditis elegans* is practically born super fertile and then very quickly loses its ability to reproduce.

Not everything weakens and becomes more likely to die as it ages. While some species grow stronger and less likely to die through the passage of time, others are practically immune to aging. Put simply, increasing feebleness and infertility with age is not a law of nature, but we humans think of it that way. On one end of the spectrum, a species can live a long time but have increasing mortality, and on the other end, a species can live a short time yet have declining mortality. In the words of the study's lead author, Owen Jones: "It makes no sense to consider aging to be based on how old a species can become. Instead, it is more interesting to define aging as being based on the shape of mortality trajectories: whether rates increase, decrease or remain constant with age." He hopes his research spurs more study in this fascinating field to help us address aging in humans.

One barrier to the study of human aging is finding appropriate models in other species that age like we do. Although old people, especially those who can make it past one hundred, may seem a logical focus for scientists, such an endeavor would move at a glacial pace. Think about it: you'd need to take seventy to eighty years or more to examine people's aging processes and know the outcome of your intervention. Not very realistic or practical. So instead, we use mice, which live only three to four years but share many of the same characteristics of our DNA and reflect many features of our aging process. From studies in mice, we've learned how genes become more or less active with age, and we can even test drugs to make mice live longer and better.

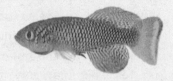

The short-lived killifish, some species of which have a life span of a couple of months and serve as excellent models for aging studies. This killifish can reach a length of about 6.5 centimeters (2.6 inches) at maturity.

Another animal that has proven very useful is the turquoise killifish. It's a rare fish indeed, found chiefly in the ponds that form during the rainy season in East Africa. Once the eggs hatch from the mud and spring to life, they grow to full size within forty days and measure about 2.5 inches. They live only a few months. But their aging resembles that of humans to a stunning degree. Like us becoming more senile as the years wear on, turquoise killifish lose their ability to learn new things. Their immune systems weaken. Their muscle mass shrinks like ours does as we age. The females become infertile. One team of researchers at Stanford has taken the study of the turquoise killifish (which owes its name partly to the slight shimmering turquoise hue on its scales) to new levels by sequencing the fish's entire genome, and in the process identifying a number of genes known to influence aging in other species, including mice and humans. They've even built molecular tools to play with the fish's genes, one of which is the same one I mentioned earlier: CRISPR. As I described, CRISPR acts like scissors to cut out pieces of DNA, literally, so they can be replaced by other pieces of DNA. Using this technique, the researchers have managed to tweak certain genes related to aging and affect how the fish age. Research like this is exciting and offers hope of finding antiaging treatments that can help us age slower and live longer. A compound, for example, that extends the life in the mighty killifish by a mere two weeks may ultimately lead to a substance that adds years to human life.

But context matters. The context of a fifty-year-old is not the same as the context of a twenty-year-old. Similarly, the context of a diabetic with asthma is not the same as that of someone with heart disease and depression. But, ideally, every context can be nurtured and cared for to slow the aging process. If this weren't true, then we wouldn't see such immense discrepancies among people of the same chronological age (the age in years) but whose respective "biological ages" are extraordinarily different. At Duke's Center for the Study of Aging and Human Development, scientists in collaboration with other institutions tracked almost a thousand New Zealanders born between 1972 and 1973 (the Dunedin Study) and calculated their "biological age" twenty years after they turned eighteen.[6] Although there's been a proliferation of age calculators lately, including websites where you can enter a few numbers and share details about your lifestyle to arrive at a "biological age" (as opposed to chronological age), we don't yet have a standardized clinical measure of biological age.

To reflect the aging process accurately, these researchers based this theoretical biological age on a wide range of parameters, measuring kidney, lung, and liver function, low-density lipoprotein (LDL, or "bad" cholesterol), dental health, metabolic and immune systems, cognitive health, and even the condition of blood vessels at the back of the eye. These tiny eye blood vessels are an established surrogate for the state of the brain's blood vessels. Eighteen biomarkers in total were tracked, the results of which were checked against tests usually given to older folks to gauge aging, including functions like coordination, muscle strength, gait, balance, and cognitive abilities.

The researchers, who examined the volunteers at age twenty-six, thirty-two, and thirty-eight, found that while the majority aged at a normal pace (one biological year for each chronological year), a few aged shockingly faster or slower.[7] In fact, the results indicated that the biological ages of the thirty-eight-year-olds ranged from twenty-eight to sixty-one years old. Some aged as much as three years within the course of just one calendar year. Those who were deemed physiologically older also looked older. And one of the more disturbing findings was that people who were aging the fastest before midlife were already showing signs of cognitive decline and brain aging, and were less physically able. People who showed accelerated aging in the biomarker tests also performed poorly on other tests.

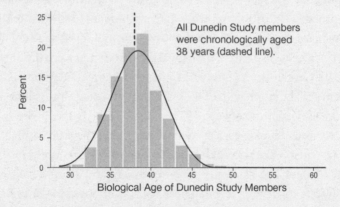

The biological age distribution of the participants of the Dunedin Study in New Zealand. The chronological age of all of the participants was 38 years.

This was among the first studies to look at young adults in the hopes of understanding why people grow old at different rates, a phenomenon we've only just begun to explore. The authors of the study, published in *Proceedings of the National Academy of Sciences* in 2015, wrote: "Our findings indicate that aging processes can be quantified in people still young enough for prevention of age-related disease, opening a new door for antiaging therapies."[8] They also stressed the importance of studying the young in searching for the secrets to prolonging healthy life, and that we "may be focused on the wrong end of the lifespan" when we look solely at people in the second half of life. Tests like the one these researchers came up with will only get more data driven, precise, and useful in the future, as biomarkers are added, dropped, and given different weights or importance. Such calculators can translate to medical savings as well. If you find out at fifty that your body is biologically behaving like a forty-year-old's, then you might not need a routine mammogram or colonoscopy as frequently as someone biologically older might.

Other, more specific calculators will also be developed and become more sophisticated. Do you know, for example, how "old" your heart is? You can find out using an online calculator developed by the National Heart, Lung, and Blood Institute and Boston University. You might be surprised to learn that your heart is not as youthful as your chronological age. In a 2015 report by officials at the Centers for Disease Control (CDC), 3 out of 4 adults between the ages of 30 and 74 in the United States were found to have a predicted "heart age" older than their actual age.[9] Specifically, men had a predicted heart age of nearly 8 years older than their chronological age; women had a heart age that was 5.4 years older. This was determined using data from the large and well-established Framingham Heart Study and involved information from more than 570,000 participants. The calculator takes into consideration various risk factors such as smoking, blood pressure, diabetes status, and weight as measured by body mass index. A riskier profile means an "older" heart.

The study also found geographic differences. Those with the "oldest" hearts live primarily in the South, with Mississippi, West Virginia, Kentucky, Louisiana, and Alabama having the highest percentage of adults with a cardiovascular age of 5 years or more over their real age. Younger hearts are found in places like Utah, Colorado, California, Hawaii, and Massachusetts. Note that people tend to have younger hearts where there are lower rates of smoking and obesity, both of which are huge risk factors for cardiovascular challenges.

The purpose of the calculator is not to discourage, but to inspire people to take steps to de-age their hearts by quitting smoking, losing weight, and considering certain drugs (e.g., blood pressure medication and statins). We know that people who calculate their heart age are more likely to try to improve their cardiovascular health, compared to those who receive only general information or who wait until their first cardiovascular event to learn about their risk factors.

As much as youth—and oldness—is a state, so is health. If we think along these lines, addressing matters of health and wellness becomes simple. Coley didn't understand why his toxins were working, and for him—and his patients—that didn't really matter. Similarly, Metchnikoff didn't understand the exact mechanism by which gut bacteria were contributing to healthy physiology. But that didn't matter, either. Both physicians observed results that benefited their patients.

It's important to maintain a perspective about your health that appreciates your body's complexity and mystery. You may never be able to understand or know everything about its inner workings or why, for example, X is said to cause Y. As I always like to emphasize, honor the human body and its relationship to disease as a complex, emergent system that you'll probably never fully comprehend. By *emergent*, I'm referring to the notion that we are more than the sum of our individual parts and even our parts' individual properties.

To understand this concept, which appears in subjects as diverse as philosophy, science, and art, consider your heart, which is obviously made of heart cells. But heart cells on their own cannot pump blood. You need the whole heart to be able to do that. The pumping property of the heart is an *emergent* property of the heart—an outcome caused by intricate interactions among smaller or simpler entities that by themselves do not exhibit such properties. Heart disease, diabetes, cancer, autoimmune disorders, and neurodegenerative ailments all reflect breakdowns in that complex system. Cancer, for instance, isn't something the body "has" or "gets"; as defined earlier, it's the result of something that the body *does* with its own cells and machinery. And this is why prevention is the most important tool in aging like an oak tree (or tortoise, take your pick). Through prevention, we tip the scales in favor of choosing what the body does today and later on. What happens to us at the end of life has its roots early in life.

Cheating Cancer and Death

The human body is tremendously resilient. When faced with illness or infection, it will adapt to preserve life. With most diseases, the body waxes and wanes alongside the progression or remission of a disease. Cancer is one of the only diseases that can be aggressive and outsmart the body's resiliency. Whatever you throw at it, the cancer gets more hostile, and there's less of a chance that it will respond to anticancer therapies. Childhood cancers, on the other hand, are usually curable. So there's a switch somewhere that distinguishes cancers that are fragile and can be conquered from those that are hardy and, ultimately, lethal. Relatively few cancers happen to people between the ages of twenty-five and fifty. Future research will likely bear out the reasons for this difference and offer some new therapies to turn deadly cancers into weak, combatable ones. Or ones that we can quarantine somehow and babysit with drugs so they don't misbehave or harm the body.

In the past I've criticized my field of medicine for its lack of progress in finding meaningful treatments that can delay the progress of cancer or prevent it entirely with proven therapies. But now we're finally seeing some hope with new technologies such as sequencing tumors and targeting cancerous growths molecularly with pills that essentially turn off the switch that makes a cell go rogue. This buys one of the most precious commodities: time. For a patient with a terminal illness, an extra few weeks or a month can be significant—especially if there's hope of a new therapy around the corner. Molecular targeting is used much more commonly now than it was when we employed it for Steve Jobs's therapy, but it doesn't work in everyone; it is currently helping about 20 to 30 percent of cancer patients, across all types of cancers. And it can be expensive, but I predict this will change as various economic forces drive costs down. To get a closer sense of how molecular targeting works, take a look at the following. This particular example is from a tumor DNA sequencing company called Foundation Medicine.[10]

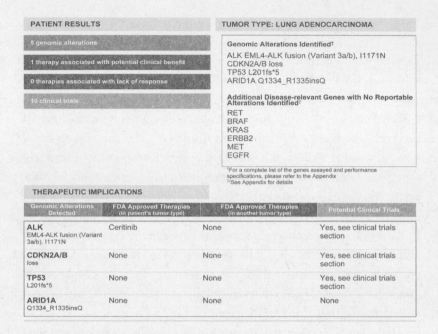

PATIENT RESULTS	TUMOR TYPE: LUNG ADENOCARCINOMA

5 genomic alterations	**Genomic Alterations Identified[†]** ALK EML4-ALK fusion (Variant 3a/b), I1171N CDKN2A/B loss TP53 L201fs*5 ARID1A Q1334_R1335insQ
1 therapy associated with potential clinical benefit	
0 therapies associated with lack of response	**Additional Disease-relevant Genes with No Reportable Alterations Identified[†]** RET BRAF KRAS ERBB2 MET EGFR
10 clinical trials	
	[†]For a complete list of the genes assayed and performance specifications, please refer to the Appendix [‡]See Appendix for details

THERAPEUTIC IMPLICATIONS

Genomic Alterations Detected	FDA Approved Therapies (in patient's tumor type)	FDA Approved Therapies (in another tumor type)	Potential Clinical Trials
ALK EML4-ALK fusion (Variant 3a/b), I1171N	Ceritinib	None	Yes, see clinical trials section
CDKN2A/B loss	None	None	Yes, see clinical trials section
TP53 L201fs*5	None	None	Yes, see clinical trials section
ARID1A Q1334_R1335insQ	None	None	None

The tumor gene sequencing report of a patient with advanced lung cancer.

This shows the results of tumor sequencing for a patient with lung cancer. These are the reports I get when I send a piece of cancerous tissue to be examined and genetically sequenced. Don't bother trying to understand the gibberish of the coding that we use to label the genes. Focus on the results: a total of five genomic mutations, or alterations in four target genes, are found related to the lung cancer in this patient.

The piece of the cancer that was used for the sequencing comes from what's called a paraffin block of tumor; it's basically a very small sliver of the cancer that was extracted from the patient and placed into a waxy material (paraffin) where it can be stored after surgery and reviewed by the pathologist before going on for genetic testing.

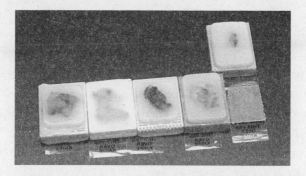

A group of paraffin (wax) blocks with pieces of tumor embedded within them.

Every cancer patient has one of these—samples of the tumor upon which the diagnosis is made. The following image is of a lung biopsy being performed. In this case, a needle is placed into the tumor to retrieve the biopsy.

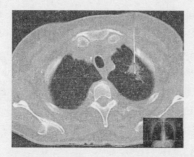

This is a CT scan image of a lung biopsy in a case of suspected lung cancer. The needle is seen on the right entering the lung mass. The small image on the lower right shows where the larger image was taken from the patient (where the line intersects the patient).

DNA is then isolated from this piece and sequenced. When DNA from the biopsied cells is compared with DNA in the patient's noncancerous cells, we can identify the changes of DNA that made it a cancer. These are the "on" switches. Now, let's go back to the sequencing results.

For one of the targets, ALK, an FDA-approved drug is available. This drug has tremendous benefit, but only in patients that have this gene altered. The good news also for the cancer sequenced here is that in addition to having at least one potential therapy to try, there are ten clinical trials this patient can also consider—opportunities to try other drugs whose effects on this type of cancer are still being tested.

Anyone can find out about all the clinical trials taking place today by going to clinicaltrial.gov and learning about which ones are still open to new patients and how to become involved if possible. Clinical trials are nothing to be afraid of; they are important in our quest to find new solutions and identify which drugs might help which individuals, even if the number of people helped is small. In the future, of course, we will get better at running trials, so that their outcomes are more meaningful for more people, and we will improve the success rate for drug development and new treatment plans. It's important to note that clinical trials of new drugs or approaches to care are done only after we've tested them in a laboratory setting using cells and animal models. The most promising treatments seen in these early experiments are then studied in people via a carefully controlled trial that follows a strict protocol over the course of multiple phases. Guidelines called eligibility criteria exist for every clinical trial; they spell out who can and cannot participate. This ensures the most reliable results, as participants must be alike in key ways—age, gender, type of condition, previous treatments, and health status. The goals of the trial's phases, depending on the questions that we're trying to answer, could be to show that a new treatment is safe, works better than an established one, or has fewer side effects than the standard therapy.

All clinical trials in the US must be reviewed by what's called an IRB, or an institutional review board. This is an independent committee of professionals including physicians, researchers, statisticians, and patient advocates whose job is to protect the rights, safety, and well-being of the subjects in the clinical trial and minimize its risks. Patients who join the trial must be fully informed and protected.

The best trials are those that are "randomized," meaning that one group receives the experimental drug and another group receives the current standard treatment. This allows us to have a way of comparing the new therapy to the usual kind. Randomization also verifies that everyone in the trial has an opportunity to get either the new treatment or the usual one. In a "double-blind study," neither the patient nor the doctor knows which treatment the patient is getting; this helps strengthen the credibility of the results by reducing the researchers' biases when they make their evaluations. If you enter a clinical trial that is randomized and double-blind, you are notified during the informed consent process, and you can then decide whether you want to participate or not.

I often get asked about placebos, as many patients who fantasize about receiving a blockbuster new drug in a clinical trial fear that they'll be allocated to the placebo group and miss out. Placebos are "dummy pills"—drugs that look exactly like the real ones being studied, but have no effect (and placebos can come in any form, including liquid and powder, so long as they mimic the experimental drug). In fact, we don't use placebos in most cancer-related clinical trials. But some trials use a placebo for a good reason: it's often the only way to know whether a new approach or drug works. In these cases, participants are told before they decide to join, during the informed consent process. And any trial can be halted at any point if one group appears to be doing significantly better than the other. This is what happened with a trial for the breast cancer drug tamoxifen in April of 1998. When doctors documented that the high-risk women in the National Cancer Institute–sponsored Breast Cancer Prevention Trial who took tamoxifen showed a 45 percent reduction in breast cancer, those who had been taking a placebo were immediately invited to switch to the active drug.

Let's go back to the genetic profile of this individual with lung cancer. It is not from a patient of mine, but I have a great many examples from my own case files that show not just the power of drugs to squash cancer cells, but the power of dosage. The following story is true, but I changed the name of the patient, whom we'll call Rick. I briefly mentioned this story in the introduction.

Rick has lung cancer—a tumor that exhibits the same altered gene called ALK, which the drug ceritinib (Zykadia) and several others can target. Initially, the tumor, which had metastasized throughout the body, responded beautifully to treatment with one of the ALK-targeting drugs. But over time, as with so many stealthy cancers, some of the cells dodged the treatments and traveled to his brain, where the cancer was growing. The cancer in the rest of the body wasn't growing and was still responding to treatment.

While discussing his case with colleagues, I wondered what I could do now to attack the cancer. My weapon wasn't reaching Rick's brain because of the blood-brain barrier, which shields the organ from outside, foreign molecules. While this "fence" was supposed to insulate the brain, in this case, it was harming the patient: it was letting cancer in while preventing the cancer drug from following it to attack. Some colleagues suggested I go from giving the drug every day to every *other* day but at a much higher dose, hoping that extra punch would overcome the blood-brain barrier and penetrate inside. Once again, I was flying blind, but I had nothing to lose. So I tried it, and it worked. At this writing, Rick is still one of the leaders of an enormous company, and he's working every day—nearly four years after his lung cancer was first diagnosed. The right drug at the right dosage can be life-saving.

Let me show you one more molecular test result from an individual with bladder cancer:

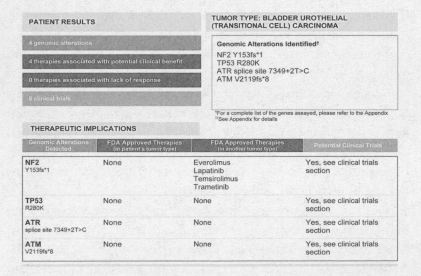

PATIENT RESULTS	TUMOR TYPE: BLADDER UROTHELIAL (TRANSITIONAL CELL) CARCINOMA
4 genomic alterations	**Genomic Alterations Identified[†]**
4 therapies associated with potential clinical benefit	NF2 Y153fs*1
0 therapies associated with lack of response	TP53 R280K
8 clinical trials	ATR splice site 7349+2T>C
	ATM V2119fs*8

†For a complete list of the genes assayed, please refer to the Appendix
ⁿSee Appendix for details

THERAPEUTIC IMPLICATIONS

Genomic Alterations Detected	FDA Approved Therapies (in patient's tumor type)	FDA Approved Therapies (in another tumor type)	Potential Clinical Trials
NF2 Y153fs*1	None	Everolimus Lapatinib Temsirolimus Trametinib	Yes, see clinical trials section
TP53 R280K	None	None	Yes, see clinical trials section
ATR splice site 7349+2T>C	None	None	Yes, see clinical trials section
ATM V2119fs*8	None	None	Yes, see clinical trials section

The tumor gene sequencing report of a patient with advanced bladder cancer.

This person has some hope from the molecular test: there are four genetic defects identified as being associated with the cancer, and for one of the mutations, four FDA-approved therapies exist that may help target it, though these drugs are FDA-approved for other types of cancer. And even though there aren't any known therapies to target three of the patient's mutations, there are clinical trials underway that he or she can investigate and potentially enter. I should point out that when a drug isn't approved by the FDA to treat one specific disease or condition, that doesn't mean a doctor cannot prescribe it and use it "off-label." To be clear, if a drug is used off-label, that doesn't necessarily mean that it's dangerous or unproven. Certain drugs are off-label only because the pharmaceutical company chose not to go through the expense and work the FDA requires to approve a drug for a specific condition or disease—especially when it comes to rare conditions that afflict only a few people.

Many of the treatments we use in cancer are in fact off-label uses of FDA-approved drugs. For example, many of the combination therapies we use to treat lymphoma, breast cancer, and colon cancer aren't FDA approved for these specific cancers. While off-label drug use can bring benefits to many patients, it isn't always paid for by insurance companies. Imagine if this person with bladder cancer got this result back from the lab and his doctor recommended a drug to treat the cancer based on the profile, but the insurance company said it won't pay, and the drug costs $100,000 or more per year. This is a common scenario in the cancer world today.

It used to be that only a small handful of new drugs for diseases emerged each year, but now new drugs are coming out routinely, even in my domain. Targeted therapies like imatinib (Gleevec) and trastuzumab (Herceptin), for example, have emerged over the past decade as standard treatments for several different types of cancer. These drugs fire at cancer cells by homing in on specific molecular changes seen primarily in those cells. And as immunotherapies also come into the picture—buying people months or sometimes years—we'll begin to see medicine enter a new phase in which cells become living drugs.

This has been called the third pillar of medicine.[11] The pharmaceuticals that arose from synthetic chemistry made up the first pillar. Then, after Genentech produced insulin in a bacterium in 1978, there was the revolution of protein drugs. Now drug companies are hoping to use our own cells as the treatment. In the case of T cells, there is tantalizing evidence that some cancers could be treated with few side effects other than a fever. And if early results hold, tests of engineered T cells in blood cancers may lead to a relatively quick FDA approval for the treatment of cancer. It could take as little as seven years, whereas the average drug takes closer to fourteen.

The other good news is that quicker access to experimental drugs will mean more people who are suffering from serious or life-threatening illnesses can potentially benefit. In 2015, the FDA moved to simplify the process for doctors to obtain such drugs, so that instead of a doctor needing one hundred hours to complete the forms necessary to apply for experimental treatments, it takes less than one hour. Not every patient who wants an experimental drug can get it. Patients are eligible when there is nothing else that can diagnose or treat their disease or condition and they cannot be enrolled in a clinical study testing the experimental drug. Risk must also be assessed, and it must be demonstrated that the probable risk from the disease exceeds the probable risk from the experimental drug. And the doctor must ensure that the manufacturer is willing to provide it. The FDA can't compel the manufacturer to dispense the drug to an individual; it simply offers guidance on how to do it. Once an application has been filed, the FDA authorizes a vast majority of requests within days or even hours.

There will, however, be challenges to address in the pharmaceutical landscape going forward, starting with pricing. We have a system that assigns a cost to each pill or infusion. The longer a patient is receiving the treatment, the higher the costs. The costs are thereby spread out over long periods. But these new treatments may be given only once, thereby making "onetime opportunities," so to speak, for pharmaceutical companies to profit. How do you assign a cost to such a treatment? No one is quite sure yet how a personalized cell therapy will be commercialized on a large scale. One day it will probably be possible, for example, to scale immunotherapies and mass-produce off-the-shelf T cells or even do genetic engineering at a patient's bedside that won't cause anyone—neither the patient nor the drug company engineering the T cells—to go bankrupt. Some labs are working with instruments to pump genetic material into cells using electricity or pressure. Others have shown they can generate T cells in a lab dish and use them to cure mice, raising the possibility of T-cell factories. For now, though, all the engineered T-cell treatments in clinical testing use a patient's own cells, and the process of creating these special cells is laborious and costly.

None of these hurdles will be impossible to overcome. They may, in fact, lead to new insights about the human body and maladies like cancer as we develop these technologies and aim to push costs down.

In 1970, Richard Peto, a British epidemiologist who helped established the importance of meta-analyses and is a leading expert on deaths related to tobacco use, introduced his namesake paradox. According to Peto's paradox, there's very little relationship between the size of an animal and cancer rates. Elephants can be eighty times the size of a human with proportionally more cells, but very rarely do they get cancer. The same goes for whales and the extinct woolly mammoths.

This seems to defy logic because the more cells an organism has, the higher the chance for mutations and resulting cancerous growth. So something else is going on to cause this phenomenon—and we finally gained some clues in 2015 when two different teams of scientists discovered that elephants' cells have 20 copies (40 alleles) of the p53 gene, which is a now-famous gene associated with protecting us from cancer. We only have one copy (2 alleles).[12] In fact, p53 has been referred to as the "guardian of the genome."[13] It's what we call a tumor suppressor gene. It has three known functions: 1) it induces DNA repair mechanisms when it senses DNA alterations from the original genome; 2) it stops cells from dividing when it detects DNA alterations, thereby allowing for more efficient DNA repair; and 3) it pushes cells to self-destruct when there are too many DNA mutations to repair. Most human tumors are associated with a mutation in one of our two alleles of p53. Loss of one of the alleles leads to Li-Fraumeni syndrome, which means more than a 90 percent lifetime risk for cancer, multiple primary tumors, and early childhood cancers. Although it isn't yet proven that those extra p53 genes make elephants cancer-resistant, further research to confirm it could lead to new drugs to mimic the effect of p53 and new ways to protect people from cancer.

I've been accused of playing inside baseball when it comes to new discoveries in medicine. I'll get excited at the smallest, most trivial of scientific findings that deserve publication in a prestigious journal but that the average person could not care less about because it's not a cure. The difference between the number of p53 genes in elephants versus humans is but one example. But what many don't realize is that these little wins—these seemingly small eureka moments and realizations— are much bigger than the sum of their parts. And they build upon one another, taking us closer to those cures we so desperately want.

Cracking Codes and Changing Conversations

Joan (pronounced Joe-ahn) Massagué Solé is the director of the Sloan Kettering Institute and chair of the Cancer Biology and Genetics Program at Memorial Sloan Kettering Cancer Center. I admire him greatly for the contributions he's made in my world of oncology. His work is proof that radical changes to the treatment of cancer that will extend the lives of millions are possible, for they are taking shape in labs the world over today. Massagué has been dubbed "the unintentional scientist"; he never thought he'd stay in America after landing here from his native Spain in 1979 to do a two-year postdoctoral fellowship at Brown University.[14] But two years later, he decided not to go back home, where he probably would have joined his pharmacist parents in their drugstore. Instead, he stuck it out to pursue more science in a country that loved to cater to his competitive streak and fierce determination.

And that perseverance paid off. He's gone down in history as the man who succeeded in understanding the code to the TGF-beta (transforming growth factor beta) pathway, an intricate and highly regulated affair that's essentially a molecular "conversation" through which cells tell one another to stop multiplying, among other actions. Since cancer is a disease of mad cellular copying, where cells don't know how to stop dividing, Massagué knew he was on to something when he began to study this important "conversation."

Growth factors in general are biological messengers that cells release into the space between one another. These chemical couriers then travel to nearby cells to deliver their message by locking on to them through a door on the surface of the cell called a receptor. But that's just the beginning in a long cascade of events whereby the message is passed to a number of different players before it culminates in the intended effect, or outcome, of the message. For a long time, we didn't know much about TGF-beta, its message, its receptor, and what happened once the details of its message got relayed. It was so complicated that even people in the field didn't bother to spend time and effort investigating it. Good thing Massagué dedicated much of his professional life to this particular "telegram," although he didn't intend for that to happen either. He found himself uniquely driven to know the whole story of TGF-beta. It became, in his words, his "playground."

A protein secreted by cells, TGF-beta has many functions in most cells, but for the most part, it controls cellular proliferation and differentiation—dictating when cells can multiply and what they will become when they grow up. It plays a role in not just cancer but also in immunity generally and a spectrum of illnesses, from the relatively mild, like asthma and diabetes, to the severe, such as heart disease, Parkinson's disease, multiple sclerosis, and AIDS. In normal cells, TGF-beta halts the cell cycle at a certain point through its signaling pathway to stop proliferation, induce differentiation, or trigger programmed cell death (apoptosis). When a cell becomes a cancer cell, however, parts of the TGF-beta signaling pathway are changed, and TGF-beta no longer controls the cell. These cancer cells are then able to multiply without any brakes.

In addition to telling the story of TGF-beta, Massagué has worked tirelessly on another characteristic of cancer that has evaded scientists for centuries: metastasis, or the process by which cancer cells exit the mothership (the tumor of origin), travel to distant tissues, and invade. Massagué's work has also been helped by the contributions of one of my mentors, Dr. Larry Norton, a breast cancer oncologist also at Memorial Sloan Kettering Cancer Center. The combination of a biologist like Massagué and a clinician like Norton has led to surprising new insights into the anatomy of cancer and its body-snatching ingenuity.

The ancient Egyptians knew about metastasis. The word owes its origins to the Greek verb for "change," *methistanai*. In the late sixteenth century, it took on a rhetorical meaning: "rapid transition from one point to another." Which is what metastasis is all about. It's still the biggest challenge in cancer—the boogeyman. If it weren't for metastasis, cancer would not be what it is today; you'd just excise the tumor like you extract a bad tooth or trim a hangnail and you'd go home. The whole point of chemotherapy and radiation after surgery is mostly to avoid or treat metastasis.

Studying metastasis isn't as easy as you might expect. Cells are not efficient at metastasis, so it's hard to find the ones that hold the key controls. Original tumors dump millions of cells every day into the bloodstream, but not all of those cells have the power to metastasize. If you die from metastatic cancer, you don't die of millions of metastases. Massagué and Norton injected into mice some cells from the tumor of a woman who had died of breast cancer. These mice were engineered to have weak immune systems that wouldn't notice the foreign cells, so their cancer would grow. Then Massagué and Norton collected the cells that traveled to the bone, which is where breast cancer cells like to go and take root. Next, the researchers took breast cancer cells that had metastasized to the mouse bones and injected those into a second group of mice. Bone tumors developed in those mice in half the time one would expect. This meant that Massagué and Norton had isolated the cellular boogeymen—the cells that hold the controls to metastasis.

Massagué and Norton's work has revealed many new facts about these offenders. Although we used to think that cells were either born with the capability to metastasize or acquire it later, we know now that cells both start out with the power to metastasize *and* gain it later. Cancer cells that leave their tumor of origin and become seeds for new tumors elsewhere in the body aren't necessarily confined to their new home. We also know now that the craftiest of circulating tumor cells can not only go out to metastasize, but can also travel back home to their tumor of origin in a process called self-seeding. Massagué and Norton performed an experiment on a mouse in which they put green-colored breast cancer cells into one breast and uncolored cells into the other. After sixty days, the green-colored cells were found in both breasts. These cancer cells are akin to scouts, and they might be transmitting important messages back to the tumor about the patient when they return.

The discovery that tumor cells are swimming in our blood has paved the way for liquid biopsies: minimally invasive blood tests that can detect cancer cells or DNA that have been shed into the bloodstream from tumors. So instead of removing pieces of tissue from the tumor itself in a traditional biopsy, doctors simply draw blood from almost all patients with metastatic cancer and isolate cancer cells. These cells can be profiled molecularly, just like the tumor biopsy I described earlier. While this is certainly much easier for the patient, most important, it also facilitates frequent monitoring of the cancer's molecular changes. This kind of technology will help us stay ahead of any cancer that is out scouting for a new address in a distant, vital organ, and allow us to change treatments as soon as we see those changes.

Massagué and his team are also credited with discovering that many of the genes that lead to metastasis work together. Activating just one or two of them doesn't achieve their goal of spreading cancer. In 2003, Massagué presented the gene combination he identified in breast cancer cells that are prone to spread to the bone. Then in 2007, he published findings on four genes that control blood vessel growth and are likely critical to the transmission of breast cancer to the lungs. Mice experiments showed that censoring these genes individually decreased the cancerous cells' ability to park themselves and proliferate in the lungs, and that deactivating them all essentially shut the tumor down. His team has also found that certain microRNAs, which are small RNA molecules found in cells that suppress gene function, are few and far between in some metastatic cells. Once again, this suggests that a brake has been turned off or released somewhere. Adding these microRNA brakes back to cells seems to turn off genes involved in cellular copying and movement. In other words, these microRNAs neutralize the bad cells' ability to spread.

Perhaps the most astounding part of these discoveries is that the drugs to flip the "off" switch in these genes and halt their activity, and thus the cancer growth, were already on the market when Massagué published his findings. And some of these drugs were not traditionally used to treat cancer and had been developed for other illnesses! One of these was celecoxib (Celebrex), a nonsteroidal anti-inflammatory that was originally approved to treat pain and inflammation often caused by arthritis. In another unrelated study that emerged in 2015, researchers discovered that a common and generic heart drug called a beta-blocker, which targets a receptor protein in heart muscle and blocks the effects of the stress hormone epinephrine, may actually prolong ovarian cancer patients' survival.[15] This underscores my belief that we may already have the vast majority of drugs we need to combat most illnesses, including cancer.

Massagué and Norton aren't the only ones demystifying cancer and deconstructing genes to find ways to fight it. Given the extent to which cancer is now understood to be influenced by drugs and even human physiology, it's hardly surprising that scientists are turning their attention to how cancer can be crushed in ways unimaginable when I was training. Biologists and clinicians at Sloan Kettering are among countless researchers adding volumes of new data in the Lucky Years. And these dedicated people will keep asking the tough questions and exploring areas of biology doctors used to shy away from.

Will Stem Cells Save the Day?

I really do believe that the cures for many of our maladies are already inside us. In addition to learning more about our molecular and genetic brakes and switches, including those among cancer cells, we're also gaining traction by discovering entirely new metrics, such as stem cells. These are unspecialized cells capable of renewing themselves through cell division. They are the body's reservoir of ground-zero cells that can develop into a distinct, specialized cell such as a muscle cell, red blood cell, or neuron (brain cell). When a stem cell divides, each new cell has the potential either to remain a stem cell or to become ("differentiate" to) another type of cell with a specific function. As adults, stem cells are largely dormant. For some reason, they are turned off and hibernate. But what if we can find ways to turn them back on and treat various ailments like never before? Such a feat might not happen solely through therapies like parabiosis, but I trust we'll find other approaches.

The world of stem-cell research is poised to expand exponentially. We have only just begun to explore their use in therapeutics and how they may one day help us stay one step ahead of disease and degeneration—without triggering cancerous growths. In 2015, Ben Dulken and Anne Brunet of Stanford University published a paper that presented an interesting question: Are we missing something when it comes to understanding the difference between how men versus women age? They wrote: "A glance at the list of the human individuals currently living over the age of one hundred ten—supercentenarians— reveals a surefire strategy for achieving such exceptional longevity: be female. Out of the fifty-three living supercentenarians, fifty-one are female. No other demographic factor comes remotely close to sex in predicting the likelihood of achieving such an advanced age."[16]

Among mammals, females in general tend to live longer than their male counterparts do. Why is this so? Theories abound, from genetic factors carried on the Y (male) chromosome and the fact men only have one X chromosome (thus potentially rendering them more susceptible to deleterious recessive traits) to the hormonal advantages in women that confer better longevity. Evolutionary hypotheses have suggested that men and women have adapted to be fit for different needs. Females put more time and effort into having and rearing children than males do, resulting in changes to DNA that may code for longevity. Of course, these ideas are difficult to test experimentally and remain conjecture. But in all the years of debating the topic, we've forgotten one important part of the equation: the male versus female stem cell.

Because one of the hallmarks of aging is the decline of stem cells' functionality, we must ask whether the aging of stem cells differs between men and women, and whether this has consequences for disease and life span. Studies thus far have shown that some stem-cell populations in females are superior to those in males thanks to estrogen, the female sex hormone. Stem cells destined to be blood cells, for example, are more abundant in female mice than in male mice, an effect that is dependent on estrogen signaling. A similar paradigm has been described in neural stem cells where estrogen increases the proliferation of these cells in a transient manner that fluctuates throughout the menstrual cycle.

Estrogen signaling is not the sole contributor to differences in stem-cell regulation between the sexes. Other studies have shown that females also exhibit increased capacity for rapid wound healing and liver regeneration, processes that are likely dependent on resident stem-cell populations. So females tend to show increased stem-cell self-renewal, regeneration potential, and in some cases, proliferation. But the big question remains: Does this tendency toward increased self-renewal in females alter the capacity of stem cells to regenerate tissues throughout aging? Does it actually influence longevity?

Do Telomeres Tell a Story?

In recent years, we've also heard a lot about telomeres, which are the strands of DNA at the ends of chromosomes. Because they protect our genetic data and make it possible for cells to divide, they've been hailed as a linchpin to health and are believed to hold some secrets regarding how we age and develop disease. But despite the initial excitement for measuring telomeres and drawing strong correlations—shorter telomeres and shorter life—the evidence has been decidedly mixed and confusing. In fact, a 2015 study in *Human Molecular Genetics,* using data from 50,000 cancer cases and 60,000 control cases, showed that the longer your telomeres were, the higher the risk for lung cancer.[17] The role of telomere length in health will be a complicated one, and it is too early now to know its meaning.

While telomere shortening has been associated with the aging process, we don't know yet whether shorter telomeres are just a sign of aging, akin to gray hair and wrinkles, or whether they actually *contribute* to aging. Those are two very different things. Once we figure out why gender can be such a factor in the aging process, it's possible we'll no longer look at telomeres in the same way, which may be reflecting how fast one is aging and not commanding the process.

Holding On to Optimism

If you've ever been to a school reunion, you've seen the difference between those who have become fat and bald before their time and the ones who look like they haven't aged a day since you last saw them. I can't tell you how many times I meet couples of the same age who look vastly different in their physical "age." And what I find most striking is that nine times out of ten, the younger-looking individual has something else that's not nearly as present in the "older" person: positivity. Optimism. An upbeat personality, a perspective that sees the glass as half full.

It's cliché, but it's true: having a positive outlook about the world and even the future of medicine is key to health. I see it every day in my practice, even among those who are prone to depression and do what they can to manage it successfully. And it's easier to be optimistic if you remember that breakthroughs are about to happen in many areas of medicine (not just oncology) that will change how you engage with doctors and how you live.

A great example of a new technology that will soon change our lives and help us to positively extend them is called near-infrared spectroscopy (NIRS). It's been around for a while in very large and expensive machines found in major corporations and labs. In simple terms, without getting into the chemistry and physics of the technology, every chemical in nature has a certain and unique profile on the electromagnetic spectrum—the range of all possible frequencies of electromagnetic radiation. This means every object has a different spot on the electromagnetic spectrum, based on the chemicals that make it up; the electromagnetic profile of any given thing is the characteristic range of electromagnetic radiation it emits or absorbs. An apple, for example, has a different profile than an apricot or an aspirin. So imagine taking a handy little device and putting it up against an object and getting an immediate readout of all the chemicals in that item. That's what you could do if you had a database of all the possible profiles.

An Israeli company has done just that, funded by a Kickstarter campaign. Their low-cost handheld tool can study a pill, for example, compare the pill's profile against a cloud database, and come back with "ibuprofen, brand Advil." Besides eliminating fake drugs, it will bring peace of mind to patients by preventing pill mix-ups. This technology could also be used to point at a plate of food and characterize how much protein, fat, and carbohydrates are in a snack or meal. Or it could analyze your urine in a toilet and tell you how well hydrated you are. The possibilities are endless, and this kind of data may prove to be more useful for real-time medicine than what's in your medical record.

Even the medicine itself will become easier to swallow. If you've ever choked on a pill that was too big, help is on the way, thanks to three-dimensional printing technologies that are revolutionizing the manufacturing of drugs. In the future, 3-D printing that helps create everything from toys and mechanical parts to new organs, biological tissues, and prosthetics will also be employed to make smaller drugs that dissolve quickly, no matter their dosage. A pharmacy of the future may just be a printer and a drawer of chemicals, where the pharmacist is able to print, on demand, any medication, just by having its chemical structure.

What gets me especially enthusiastic about the Lucky Years is that we're encountering innovations and revelations, when we least expect them, that put past headlines to shame. In December 2014, for example, I did a segment for CBS *This Morning* about "the end of antibiotics" and the coming crisis of lethal superbugs that are totally resistant to all of the antibiotics in our arsenal. The British prime minister David Cameron had just released a report he had commissioned, warning that if antimicrobial resistance was not controlled, it could compromise the advances of modern medicine and swallow up to 3.5 percent of the global economy.[18] The report went on to state that increasing rates of drug-resistant infections could lead to the death of some 10 million people and cost upwards of $100 trillion by 2050.

Currently, drug-resistant bacteria infect at least 2 million people a year in the United States and kill 23,000. In 2014, the World Health Organization warned that such infections were happening all over the world, and that drug-resistant strains of many diseases were emerging faster than new antibiotics could be developed to fight them. Compounding the problem is the fact that many drug companies have stopped trying to develop new antibiotics so they could focus on other, more profitable types of drugs.

We blamed the antibiotic-resistant strains on human invention and profligate use of antibiotics in medicine and livestock. But just in the past year, we've realized that the capacity to resist antibiotics might be a natural part of bacteria's evolutionary history. Antibiotics actually come from bacteria, which produce them to protect themselves from other bacteria so that they can effectively compete for limited food and other resources. So developing resistance to other bacteria's antibiotics would make sense as a defensive maneuver. A 2014 study revealed dozens of species of bacteria in a four-million-year-old cave that are resistant to both natural and synthetic antibiotics.[19] Such a finding supports a growing understanding that antibiotic resistance is as old as bacteria themselves. It's natural and hardwired in the microbial gene pool.

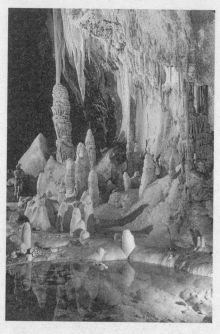

A photo from the depths of Lechuguilla Cave in New Mexico, a place isolated from human contact until very recently. This is where researchers found dozens of antibiotic-resistant bacteria and identified many of the mechanisms for antibiotic resistance in nature.

"The end of antibiotics" was an unnerving, chilling segment to produce, to say the least; it seemed so realistic and doomsdayish at the time. But no less than a month later, I was back on the morning news again, this time applauding a group of Northeastern University researchers who'd found a new method to extract bacteria that live in dirt to yield a powerful new antibiotic.[20] In these newly identified bacteria from a grassy meadow in Maine (that could only be grown when the bacteria were cultured in dirt!), a compound called teixobactin was discovered that could cure severe superbug infections. Best of all, the drug works in a way that makes it highly unlikely that bacteria will become resistant to it. Moreover, the method developed to make the drug has the potential to lead us to a treasure chest of other natural compounds to fight infections—molecules that were previously beyond our reach because the microbes that produce them could not be grown in the laboratory, as no one had yet tried to grow bacteria in a laboratory with dirt. All of a sudden, the doomsday scenario had changed, from one discovery! As for dealing with the extravagant use of antibiotics, I trust we'll find alternatives to how we treat livestock, as well as develop an over-the-counter test for humans, similar to a pregnancy test, to determine whether they are infected with bacteria to begin with. Then they can decide which course of treatment is best.

My whole point in highlighting the example of discovering new antibiotics where we least expect them is to show that the news, especially in health circles, can change in an instant. Just when we hear horrible news that deflates our hope for a better, healthier future, another piece of news trumps it. Which is why holding on to optimism is important. Every laboratory is a beacon of hope; every medical conference is a meeting of possibility. People distrust Big Pharma, but it is where much of the good news comes from.

Optimism will help you choose how you age, but to fully enjoy the Lucky Years, you must learn how to use the technology that will help you take control of your health. Don't be afraid of this process. Get comfortable with gadgetry and terminology. It's like the difference between going out to dinner every night versus using your own kitchen at home and learning how to cook. You can make all your meals, and it starts to feel powerful, and you then patronize restaurants (i.e., go to the doctor) for something special (i.e., analyzing health data). Technology can help ensure compliance. In the past, doctors took on the role of being the scolding parent. They put people back on the straight and narrow. But we can use technology to remind ourselves what to do and to compel us to change our behavior.

Most of us ignore the health care system in America until we have a problem with it, be it fighting a claim, dealing with poor service, or addressing a misdiagnosis. The passage of the Affordable Care Act left many wondering just how much it would improve the system and at the same time lower costs. The law is supposed to "put consumers back in charge of their health care," but I know that many don't feel this has been realized yet, at least not in the way they imagined when the law was being initially discussed and drafted. The problem is that unless we as individuals help change the system, we won't see a vast improvement in our system.

I'm not here to dissect the Affordable Care Act or offer advice on which plan to choose. What I do want to do, however, is show you how to participate in the system like never before so you can rest assured that your doctor's visit a decade from now will be what it should be. Clearly, we all want the system to be characterized not only by cost-effectiveness, but also by the ability to prolong and improve the quality of our lives. And to achieve this goal, we need to take charge of the system today.

Now, that may seem like an incredibly lofty, possibly even unrealistic goal. How do we assume responsibility for the system? How do we improve something that seems so complicated, amorphous, and unyielding? Well, let me start by presenting what a future doctor's visit should look like, as this will help you prepare and, in turn, begin to help you choose how you age.

CHAPTER 3

The Future You

How Your Small Data in the Context of Big Data Will Save You

He who studies medicine without books sails an uncharted sea,
but he who studies medicine without patients does not go to sea
at all.

—Sir William Osler

Anyone who has gone through medical school or read up on the history of medicine has come across the name Sir William Osler. Fondly known as the father of modern medicine (second only to Hippocrates), Osler was one of the four founding professors of Johns Hopkins Hospital who revolutionized the teaching of medicine. When he arrived at Hopkins in 1888 as physician in chief, he was already a well-known doctor and somewhat famous clinical teacher. Among his most endearing lessons was his use of alliteration to help his students retain information. The "Four F's," for example, could result in typhoid fever: fingers, food, flies, and filth. His landmark textbook about internal medicine, *The Principles and Practice of Medicine*, was published in 1892 and remains continually updated to this day.

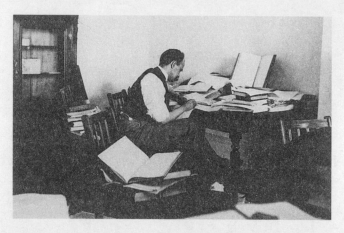

A photo of Sir William Osler writing his textbook, *The Principles and Practice of Medicine*, in the room of his chief resident, Hunter Robb, in the Billings Building at the Johns Hopkins Hospital. Osler had asked to "borrow" the room for an hour from Dr. Robb to write his masterpiece, but ended up taking over the room completely for six months.

Short and wiry, with a handlebar mustache to boot, he always dressed in three-piece suits topped with a silk bowtie. And Osler was as much renowned for his practical jokes as he was for his doctoring and teaching. In fact, "Osleriana"—language from his written works—still appears frequently in the *Journal of the American Medical Association*, as a reminder of his wise and common tidbits.

Perhaps Osler's greatest contribution to medicine and to health care in general was to require that students learn by example—from seeing and talking to real patients. He established the first medical residency program, an idea that would eventually spread across the Western world and become the main system by which teaching hospitals operate. Even today, when you walk into a teaching hospital, much of the medical staff is composed of doctors in training. Osler also initiated another tradition in medical school by getting his students to the bedside early in their training. Rather than spend the majority of their time sitting in a lecture taking notes, third-year students mastered how to take patient histories, perform physicals, and order lab tests to examine various bodily fluids. He once said he hoped that his tombstone would read only, "He brought medical students into the wards for bedside teaching." (Osler's body was cremated; his ashes rest in the Osler Library of Medicine at McGill University, his alma mater.)

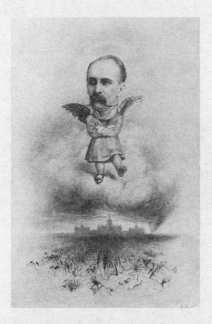

A caricature of William Osler that shows him elevated to a holy status as he sweeps away disease. The title, *The Saint—Johns Hopkins Hospital*, is a play on Osler's frequent reference to the hospital as "the St. Johns." The caricature was done in 1896 by Max Broedel, a renowned medical illustrator.

When I think back to my own medical training, I can't imagine what my education would have been like had I not had the opportunity to learn by hands-on experience with my mentors and their patients at the bedside. It's the kind of education you just can't get from listening to a lecture in an auditorium, even with the best visuals or wheeling in a mock patient. After completing my medical degree at the University of Pennsylvania, I went on to the Osler Medical Housestaff Training Program, as it's called, at Johns Hopkins Hospital. I remember the experience so well. On my first day, I was handed several pairs of white polyester pants. These would be part of my uniform, along with the quintessential short white coat of the first-year resident. The polyester made sure that bodily fluids would roll right off. My pockets were packed with the essentials: a cheat sheet on antibiotic dosing, a quick guide to all medical diseases, a stethoscope, a reflex hammer, no fewer than five pens, a code pager, and another pager that snapped to my belt. Walking the halls in my regalia, I felt a little like Rambo. I also carried stacks of notecards that kept track of certain patients and kept me on my toes for when I'd be quizzed by one of the senior doctors.

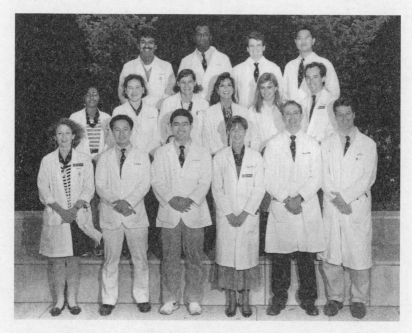

My Osler medicine residency team at Johns Hopkins Hospital in Baltimore in 1992, my first year practicing medicine. I am in the second row, far right.

Every Friday at 8:00 a.m. sharp, we medical students sat row by row in the famous Hurd Hall. The most senior physicians sat with pride in the first row. We male medical interns wore our blue Osler ties with the word *Aequanimitas* written on them. The women wore their

Osler scarves emblazoned with the same word. It was the Osler motto. The term means "imperturbability," a quality Osler felt was of utmost importance for a good physician. In his essay addressed to graduating students of the University of Pennsylvania in 1889, "Aequanimitas," Osler further defined this concept as "coolness and presence of mind under all circumstances, calmness amid storm, clearness of judgment in moments of grave peril." At these weekly events, a patient would be presented onstage, examined, and questioned briefly in front of the whole audience. Questions would rain down from the audience, and lab results would be revealed. Then a physician would give a well-studied and rehearsed lecture on the disease in question.

The power of Osler's teaching philosophy was that it brought context to his medical students. He yanked students from the confines of their two-dimensional books of information and pushed them to see the narrative in the real, three-dimensional world of working with patients, listening to their stories, watching their illnesses, and following their treatments. He changed not only how they were learning, but also *what* they were learning.

Now, why am I telling you all this history about someone who has nothing to do with your health in the future? Because there's a lot we all can learn from Osler, whether we're doctors or dancers. Nothing can replace the impact of what we see, hear, feel, smell, touch, and perceive in the tactile world of communicating with living people. Just think of the difference between reading a book about how to drive a car and actually driving one, or listening to someone telling you about the taste of a decadent chocolate cake and actually tasting one. Indeed, reading and lecturing provide knowledge, but they often lack valuable context to make those lessons come to life and be truly useful.

Which is why defining your own personal context in your microcosmic world will help you reap the benefits of modern technology and live better. Bring a little bit of Oslerian mentality to your personal health care. Now let me tell you what that looks like, starting with a basic lesson in context.

Matters of Context
(Or, How Everyone Is Right!)

What's the best diet? Is gluten that bad for you? Are probiotics help-ful? Are mammograms and colonoscopies necessary by a certain age, no matter what? Do you really have to be taking a baby aspirin daily for the rest of your life? What blood mercury level is safe? What kind of exercise will melt away your belly fat? Do plastics and cell phones cause cancer? When is the ideal time for you to go to bed so you wake up feeling vibrant?

Answer: It depends.

In the summer of 2014, I had the opportunity to travel with my family on safari in Africa. It was an amazing, unforgettable experience. A dream trip of mine. It taught me so much about this beautiful part of the world and its disparate cultures, but it also taught me a lot about myself and where I'd gone wrong in my thinking. In the past, I've talked a lot about the importance of using the best scientific data to know what you should be doing daily to live longer. Two of my biggest recommen-dations for people over forty, which have become points of contention for many opponents in debates with me, are taking a daily baby aspirin and considering the use of statins.

This latter suggestion is the one that caused the most stir, and it continues to get me into trouble with people who think statins are a poison to the body. Indeed, they can have unpleasant side effects in some individuals, which is precisely why they aren't for everyone. But a truth remains: multiple high-profile and rigorously controlled large studies have shown that their use can dramatically reduce the incidence of heart attack and stroke and, due to their powerful effects lowering inflammation in the body, they reduce total mortality.

Contrary to popular wisdom, statins are well tolerated in people who are the ideal candidates to take them. And most of the criticisms against statins are based solely on a philosophical aversion to them. But today I admit that I could be okay with their philosophies to some degree. Why? For starters, let me share what my African guide told me when

I asked him about how he protects himself against malaria, an illness that's endemic to his environment. What he said to me got me thinking differently: "I don't take antimalarial pills because I don't want to take them indefinitely."

Malaria is a rare but life-threatening blood disease caused by a parasite that is transmitted to humans by the *Anopheles* mosquito. It's preventable and curable but continues to plague many parts of the world. Most malaria cases and deaths take place in sub-Saharan Africa, but Latin America, Asia, and, to a lesser extent, the Middle East and parts of Europe are also affected. In 2014, ninety-seven countries and territories had ongoing malaria transmission. The complexity of the malaria parasite has evaded efforts to make a vaccine against it, though many have been in development and ones that have shown the most promise offer only partial protection that declines over time.

The majority of deaths occur among children living in Africa. Although antimalarial measures have dramatically decreased the risk of getting malaria worldwide, a child still dies every minute from the illness in Africa. Before my family and I arrived, we had been taking antimalarial medications for a couple of days and would continue to do so for a week upon return to the United States. But these drugs don't come free of side effects, and I can't imagine taking them forever if I were living in an African village where malaria is rampant.

My guide explained to me how he'd gotten used to the constant threat of the disease and that he took the right precautions every day to prevent being bitten by the mosquitoes. He wore shirts with long sleeves and pants, slept in a mosquito-free setting, and used insect repellent. Even the antimalarial drugs themselves aren't 100 percent effective and must be combined with these basic protective measures. For my guide, strategies that don't involve ingesting drugs were enough, and so far, so good. He also had faith that if he contracted malaria, he'd be able to recover with proper treatment.

This dialogue reminded me of similar conversations I've had with people who tell me they "don't want to take a statin forever," or some such. While they appreciate the preventive power of such a measure, at the same time, they don't want to commit their bodies to relying on a daily drug for the rest of their lives for prevention's sake. Obviously, if they need a drug to help manage or treat a condition, that's one thing. But to take a drug simply to lower a certain risk factor in a sea of many unrelated risk factors, that's another thing entirely. Part of me respects this perspective now, and it's one of the messages I may have gotten wrong in my previous book.

When I returned home from Africa, this new perspective shined a light on a lot of other aspects to practicing medicine and helping people navigate their health choices. I started walking around thinking *Everyone is right!* and it was liberating. For example, all diets and supplement recommendations are correct *in the right context*. And that's the difference between being right and wrong. Context eliminates the need to reduce everything down to good or bad, healthy or unhealthy, virtue or vice. As I said earlier, there is no "right" answer in health decisions—though a lot of people think they are right and try to foist their righteousness on others. Rather, there are several right answers, and probably a few really bad ones for most people. To repeat: you have to do what's right *for you*, based on your personal code of values, health circumstances, and tolerance for risk, in consultation with your own physician. Of course, this kind of informed choice demands that you be as knowledgeable about your health status and treatment options as possible, which is what you'll achieve in the Lucky Years.

The Doctor Will See You (and Your Data) Now

Today, when you go to the doctor for a wellness checkup, you make an appointment far in advance and then visit the doctor's office to get your data collected, including blood pressure, weight, and other routine lab tests. The only preparation you make beforehand is probably mental: organizing any questions you might have for your doctor and trying not to feel nervous about the visit. Several days after your appointment, someone in your doctor's office calls you back with the results of any tests or lab work that was performed. Sometimes no one even bothers to call you if everything comes back as "normal."

A future doctor's visit, on the other hand, will be all about putting the data collected into context so you can know what's best for you. You won't go there to collect data. Instead, you will go in *with* your data. Some examples that I foresee: A week prior to your appointment, you will mail a biochip to your doctor's office that contains a drop of blood from a finger prick that can be analyzed. Your smartphone and other portable devices, some of which will be wearable like watches or bracelets, will be equipped with all sorts of technologies to measure various features about your health. They can listen to your heart and send an EKG to your doctor, as well as transmit the sounds of your heart to a sound cloud to compare and analyze against people who share the same age and lifestyle. They can perform a retinal scan and detect an impressive array of potential problems, from high blood pressure and diabetes to cancer. The data will also have context. What did your blood pressure do when you were upset after a telephone call? How high did your pulse rate go with exercise? How much did you move in the past twenty-four hours? What was your heart rate variability, which is a marker for stress?

If you're pregnant, those routine prenatal exams will also be transformed through technology, allowing you to monitor the health of your baby all on your own and send data to your obstetrician for review and/or discussion. You won't even need to undergo an invasive amniocentesis or chorionic villus sampling to examine the chromosomes of the fetus and make sure everything is copacetic. Instead, a small sample of blood will reveal everything a mother-to-be would want to know about her developing baby—and even more about herself. A new type of prenatal test widely available and intended to find genetic flaws in a fetus through the mother's blood can also reveal previously undiagnosed cancer in the mother. This was an unexpected finding by scientists who were looking for a less invasive way to test a fetus—another example of pure serendipity.

With all these innovations, your doctor won't have to spend much time collecting your information during your appointment. He or she will sit there with you and devise a game plan based on the data you provided before stepping foot in the office. The doctor can actually review the details and think about it before you arrive. Should you need any additional testing performed in light of your data, you can get it done right there—you won't have to drive somewhere else or make another appointment two weeks later. In the future, medical centers will be one-stop shopping. Now that's real-time medicine.

The whole notion of even going to the doctor when you are sick may change. If you think about it, it actually doesn't make much sense. When you don't feel well, you have to drive to an office and sit in a waiting room with others who may not like your contagious runny nose. In fact, there are now several start-up companies with doctors on call to come to your house on a moment's notice, so you can get medical assistance at home. In the future, your wellness checkups will be opportunities for you to interact with your doctor when you are well so you can exchange information and come up with a plan. And when you're sick, you'll also be able to call your doctor, with whom you'll already have a strong relationship, and seek advice for dealing with your current problem. Although technology does allow us to keep a certain distance today, the value of interaction between you and your doctor cannot be overstated.

Those old-fashioned house calls I mentioned are part of the rapidly growing field of telemedicine, which promises to bring doctors and nurses to you rather than you having to travel to their offices or enter an ER for care. In some cases, it entails live video consultations with board-certified doctors, available twenty-four hours a day, who can offer advice, prescribe medicine, and suggest follow-up care. Telemedicine will probably never entirely replace the standard doctor's office visit, but it will definitely have a role in the Lucky Years. With telemedicine, people in rural or remote areas, or those with disabilities or serious, chronic illness, can connect with specialists on a moment's notice. If going to the doctor's office is very difficult, follow-up visits can be made by video, eliminating the stress of travel. A nurse can communicate with patients regularly to answer questions or to ensure compliance with prescriptions and recommendations. And now, with the technology available, data can be collected and shared with the doctor during the telemedicine encounter. Some small towns have installed kiosks where patients can enter and have their vitals signs checked while talking with a doctor at a distant major university. All of this will help to achieve the best outcome if used correctly.

I realize that there's already some debate about whether doctors will want to deal with copious amounts of data provided by the patient, but that data ultimately helps reduce errors. Not all data is equal, but with enough data, error goes away. Measuring your blood pressure at noon in the doctor's office is one piece of data, but imagine coming in with three months' worth of data. Measuring it at night, early in the morning, after a disturbing phone call, and when you are relaxed with a glass of wine. It's a statistical fact that more data means less room for error. You may have missed the time of day when your blood pressure spikes if you only measured it once in the doctor's office. The slope, or the trend, in your data is more illuminating than a single data point. And the amount of data doesn't have to be overwhelmingly large; the basics will suffice.

Even though your doctor today won't be expecting you to arrive with a record of your patterns and data since your last visit, it helps to get into the habit of creating the documentation. Start to gather information now. Remember, the trends in data over time yield the most insightful information. The more you can collect and store, the more you will know about what to do in the future. I would even suggest that in the near future you should start to store your plasma (the part of a blood sample with all of the proteins); blood banks can freeze plasma that's stable for up to twenty years. This will allow you, in the future, to go back and compare your current condition with your data from the past, with methods that haven't yet been developed today.

An example: Let's say you develop a relentless cough in 2025 and your doctor orders a chest X-ray. On the X-ray is a 0.5-cm nodule. It could be scar tissue from a previous infection or it could be cancer. Presently, the only way to determine the diagnosis is to stick a needle in it for a sampling or remove it entirely and examine it under the microscope. This is pretty major surgery, but tens of thousands are done every year in the name of "just in case." In the future, we will have a blood test that can distinguish between cancer cells and normal cells, but it probably will require a baseline. What that means is that you'll have a baseline profile of your blood that tells you everything is fine. So once something like a mass is detected, you can consult your baseline to see if anything has changed and treat accordingly. If a certain increasing value that indicates cancer crops up, it probably means you need to take out the nodule. If the blood test has been stable for a decade, then there's no reason to worry. This will happen time and time again for each potential disorder. The tests of the future depend on context—what is going on in you today compared with what has happened in the past. By having a tube of blood stored annually, you will be able to go back to the past. Right now doing so is not routine, but I imagine this will be standard in your future annual checkup.

Aggregate Data Sets Will Save You

The other key element to this new type of visit to the doctor is that all of your data can go into a centralized database, which will create a profile of you compared to others with similar features. That database can give you advice about what to do based on your information and what you might expect to happen, much in the way you'd plug a computer into a car to diagnose the mechanical issues. Now, that's an oversimplified analogy, for a human body is much more complex than a car, but it nonetheless makes a good point: like diagnosing major problems with a car (not the exterior scratches and worn seats), the body's chief systems and fundamental physiology can be similarly evaluated (but not the arteries and underlying genetic vulnerabilities). General readouts can have value, and lead the way for further analyses.

To bring in some simple examples, imagine being able to learn, based on your unique biology within the context of a gigantic database, what to eat (or not eat) to avoid migraines, balance your blood sugar, and lose extra weight without classic dieting; when to stop consuming caffeine during the day lest you sleep poorly; what time of day is ideal for you to be outside or to break a sweat; whether or not you can benefit from any particular medications without side effects; why you wake up routinely at 3:10 a.m. and how to stop that cycle; which songs synchronize with your heart rate; when to go for a walk or otherwise engage in a stress-reducing activity because it's the time of day when your stress levels peak; and how much you should be worried about your levels of inflammation. You'll be able to leverage associations made by virtue of aggregate data sets.

So if you're a thirty-six-year-old female who played soccer in your youth but smoked until you were thirty, you'll be able to compare your health profile with others who've engaged in similar behaviors. And not only will your DNA be part of your data, but also the dynamic conversations that are taking place in your body that can be detected through a variety of measurements, from basic hormones that fluctuate through the day to the proteins found in your blood that follow a pattern and may, for instance, indicate a heightened risk for X or the need to treat Y.

Proteomics, the study of the body's proteins, is a rapidly expanding new field at the center of some of the research I'm conducting. We're exploring how proteins compose the body's language, and ultimately shape the language of health. Proteomics allows us to eavesdrop on that cellular conversation, which can inform better ways to prevent and treat disorders and diseases. Unlike your relatively static DNA, your proteins are incredibly dynamic. They change minute by minute in your body depending on what's going on internally. I can't tell from sequencing your DNA if you've just had a cocktail, what kind of foods you like to eat, when you last flexed some serious muscle, how well you slept last night, or if you are under a lot of stress. But your proteins, on the other hand, can tell. They can speak on your body's behalf, divulging information that's hard to find elsewhere. Through proteomics, I can start to look at and measure the "state" of your body. And it's that thirty-thousand-foot view that allows me to take in the whole picture, at a moment in time. DNA, while powerful and revelatory in its own right, cannot do this.

Some of the other exciting research I'm involved with entails overlaying health records from millions of people with variables such as the weather and news events. Think about examining, for example, what happens to kids who were born during the week Hurricane Sandy swept over the eastern seaboard of the United States. That one environmental impact alone could have had health consequences.

Stephen J. Elledge is a professor of genetics at Harvard Medical School and Brigham and Women's Hospital in Boston. His research is leading to tools for tracking patterns of disease in different populations. His work is ultimately helping us to understand the differences between the young and the elderly, as well as people from various parts of the world. A test he's recently developed, for example, could be used to find out whether viruses, or the body's immune response to them, have a hand in chronic diseases, including cancer. This test, called VirScan, requires just a drop of blood and can broadcast nearly every virus a person has been exposed to throughout life, past and present. First reported about in the journal *Science* in 2015, VirScan can currently identify more than a thousand strains of viruses from 206 species, which reflects the entire human "virome," or all the viruses known to infect humans, from the common cold to HIV.[1] The test works by detecting antibodies, which are the body's defense mechanisms against an invader. These are highly specific proteins the immune system manufactures to combat germs such as viruses. And once you are exposed to a virus and make an immune response to it, the antibodies stay around and provide a "record" that you were exposed to that virus.

The application of this type of test will be staggering. We will be able to generate all kinds of data from documenting people's exposures to disease. Some have compared this technology to the development of the electron microscope, which allowed us to have more resolution at the micro level and "see" things previously invisible. One application, for example, will be mapping out historical and current patterns of disease and seeing how certain diseases are affected by the type of antibodies a person has. We've long suspected that viruses may contribute to chronic ailments such as heart disease, asthma, and autoimmune diseases, the latter of which are characterized by a glitch in the immune system whereby it produces antibodies that mistake a person's own cells for foreign invaders and attack them.

There's a lot we still don't know about the relationship between, say, overcoming a flu bug and being diagnosed with type 1 diabetes or multiple sclerosis later on. But no such viruses or antibodies have ever been identified in terms of these diseases, and the research in this realm has been tricky. To look for them, we've had to single out suspect viruses and test for them individually. But with a test like VirScan, we can look at the big picture and establish Big Data to find correlations between certain viral infections and future risk of diseases. For example, an infection from virus X leads to higher risk for illness Y later in life. Or maybe those antibodies you develop as a result of that infection will *protect* you from certain ailments. The test can thus be used to shed light on an individual's risk factors and inform future health decisions. The technology might even help answer questions about cancer, which operates differently in different people. Perhaps the reason lies in which antibodies a person has, and when they developed, which in turn affects an individual's response to treatment and drugs such as chemotherapy.

The best part about this test is that it's inexpensive (about $25) and can be done in a matter of hours. This is one-stop shopping that should become part of your annual checkup so you can be as proactive as possible. And its utility will go up exponentially the more the test is deployed and the larger the database becomes.

Data mining for disease patterns won't always have to rely on bodily fluids. There will be lots of opportunities to find connections in our complex biology from even the most uncomplicated observations. Case in point: In 2014, it was discovered that artificial sweeteners wreak havoc on the body, disrupting its microbial inhabitants,[2] known collectively as the microbiome (a subject I'll cover in the next chapter). That, in turn, can affect metabolism and blood sugar balance. Although it was exploring the microbiome that finally gave us this insight, we could have known years ago about the relationship between drinking diet soda and increased risk for diabetes had another type of database been already in place to collect the information. Such a huge finding could have come from simply knowing what people buy and consume (lots of products made with artificial sweeteners) and their health profiles (lots of insulin resistance and diabetes).

For another example, consider the 2015 headline that probably caused some panic in people who take heartburn drugs that use proton pump inhibitors (PPIs) such as esomeprazole (Nexium), omeprazole (Prilosec), and lansoprazole (Prevacid). It said that these drugs, many of which are now available over the counter, can increase your risk of a heart attack up to 21 percent regardless of whether or not you have a preexisting heart condition. The beauty of this conclusion is that it came from the simplest of data mining. Researchers at Houston Methodist and Stanford University analyzed 16 million clinical documents from some 2.9 million patients.[3] That's how they traced a connection between people who were prescribed common antacids with PPIs and the chance of having a heart attack. The research was conducted after a report came out in 2013 in the journal *Circulation* that showed how PPIs could potentially lead to long-term cardiovascular disease on a molecular level: they change the lining of blood vessels.[4] Interestingly, patients who were prescribed another type of antacid that contains what are called H2 blockers had no increased likelihood of heart attack.

Antacids that contain PPIs are most often prescribed for digestive system issues, including gastroesophageal reflux disease (GERD). According to the FDA, 1 in 14 Americans has taken proton pump inhibitors, among the most commonly used drugs in the United States. So the results of this study are alarming, but keep in mind that they reflect an association—not causation. The people who take PPIs and experience heart trouble could have other health challenges that compound the problem, such as obesity, high blood pressure, and underlying genetic risk factors. Nevertheless, culling this kind of information from Big Data is part of our brave new world of medicine. It gives us more knowledge to consider in taking care of ourselves.

Let me give you one more example, one that's already in action and changing the lives of millions. Just a few years ago, the University of Nottingham developed an app called MyBabyFace with the help of the Bill & Melinda Gates Foundation. The problem: global infant mortality remains high at 22 per 1,000 live births—especially in countries where high-tech ultrasounds and skilled physicians are not readily available. The majority of these deaths occur because of bad math; it's not easy calculating an accurate age for babies being born at an unknown gestation. Consequently, premature babies are not identified in a timely fashion, and we often miss the opportunity for simple, low-cost interventions that help avoid the complications related to being born premature, such as hypothermia. The MyBabyFace app leverages the power of crowdsourcing. Parents across the world upload a photo of their baby's feet, face, and ears as well as the gestational age. The current purpose of the app is simply to collect data, and the hope is to develop a database to make it easier to judge a child's time in the womb. Another app, Neogest, uses the depth of foot wrinkles and the roundness of the eyes as clues for gauging a baby's degree of prematurity.

The Google Effect

What makes a data-mining tool like Google so brilliant is that it's a constantly evolving, giant cataloging system—a way of organizing all the information on the internet. In the computer world, we call a data structure that holds enormous amounts of data coded in a way that allows one to quickly search and retrieve information a hash table. But Google does even better than, say, the hash table used by a massive library to arrange, store, and track books. Every time somebody searches the site, Google gets better at returning results, and the site grows ever stronger and more powerful. This kind of power will come into the health realm in the Lucky Years; there will be a hash table for genomics, proteomics, environmental factors (like living next to a freeway), lifestyle habits (like eating Paleo or smoking), as well as medical conditions (like being diabetic and allergic to shellfish). Every day I treat patients similar to the ones I saw the prior week; yet I am not improving the care I give or my recommendations based on knowledge culled from previous patients, because the system is not set up for that. But it will be soon. The power of the "Google" data approach is that my care going forward will improve with every patient I treat; the database will have increasingly more information upon which to base decisions, so that my patients and I can make better ones. A colossal amount of data is being collected: it's been estimated that as much data is now generated in just two days of 2015 as was generated from the beginning of civilization until 2003.

Here's a good question: Who will host and manage all of this data, some of which is highly sensitive? A plan needs to be put forward to establish a new nonprofit entity that will host all of this data and keep it secure and anonymous. This data is a major world resource and needs to be safeguarded and kept free of biases that government and for-profit companies can bring, and which can result in abusing the database for purposes of discrimination or, worse, blackmail. We need only one host so that the database can be large enough to yield answers.

My clinic, for example, and eleven others across the country have teamed up with the IBM supercomputer known as Watson, which is being trained to analyze the genetic data from a patient's cancer and search the scientific literature to help guide treatments for this patient. As the artificial-intelligence, "cognitive" computer gets more information and learns about matching patients to treatments, Watson helps us realize the goal of truly personalized medicine. The *Washington Post* summarized the hope perfectly: "And best of all, Watson will continue to learn on the job as it hunts for appropriate oncology treatments. That means that Watson will gain in value and knowledge over time, based on previous interactions with medical practitioners. The more that participating institutions use Watson to assist clinicians in identifying cancer-causing mutations, the more that Watson's rationale and insights will improve."[5]

At one time, we were afraid to have our financial info online or use a computer to transfer money and store our financial data. Now we barely think twice about doing it. There are tools and assurances built into the system. The same needs to and will happen with health data. And we'll be able to move from doctor to doctor without repeating tests or worrying about where our records are and whether they are safe. In cases of emergency, we'll be able to quickly and effortlessly access our entire health record to optimize our care—especially if we are in dire straits and an ER physician needs to know, for instance, if we're allergic to a medication he's about to administer.

When a group of banks created a member-owned association in 1966 to revolutionize how payments could be processed without relying on traditional checks and cash, MasterCard financial services corporation was born. But think about what this company, and other banking companies, have had to overcome to make their product work in the market. They've had to establish rules for authorization; standardize the billing process; establish rules for international currency exchange; put in place guidelines and procedures to minimize fraud and other abuses; and handle marketing, security, and legal aspects to running a worldwide organization. And now they have to keep up with the increasingly hackable digital world where thieves, embezzlers, and pirates are lurking invisibly everywhere. But the financial services corporations nonetheless still work, and we consumers and debtors continue to trust and rely on them. Just think about how much more efficient the financial services industry is today—and how much easier your life is—thanks to credit cards, digital payments, and being able to view all of your money data online at the click of a mouse.

It's hard to imagine what life would be like without this system. In ten to twenty years, we will be saying the same thing about access to our health data and the data of anonymous others that adds context to our own. You check your messages today like clockwork, probably, and tomorrow you'll be similarly checking things like your blood sugar levels or heart rate using the tools available to you through handy portable devices including your phone. In the Lucky Years, your smartphone will be an incredibly powerful diary of your life that can inform your health decisions, sometimes at a moment's notice. Ultimately, this facilitates the management of disease in real time rather than around scheduled doctor's visits, allowing for quicker access to help or quicker adjustment of treatments to resolve the problem. One area in particular where this is sorely needed today is the realm of mental health. And help is on the way.

A Personal Diagnostician and Therapist in Your Pocket

Several phone apps in production promise the ability to diagnose clinical depression with exceptional accuracy. They'll even be able to detect days when you're just feeling moody or extra anxious but aren't necessarily depressed. Indeed, your phone will be able to turn into a virtual personal therapist and tell you when you seem gloomy by measuring vocal tone, tracking how much you text, and using facial recognition technology to gauge levels of stress. It will even be able to give you a pep talk to calm your anxiety. Other apps in production promise to detect signs of other mental disorders including forms of dementia. This is also possible by evaluating speech patterns and spotting vocal differences between adults aging normally and those with signs of degenerative brain conditions.

Such technology enables everyone to develop a built-in buddy system. If your friend knows via the app that you are feeling blue, he or she can act to help. At the same time, you will have a record of feeling down over time. Right now we have data only about what you remember when you are in your doctor's office. By having lots of data over time, patterns and associations can be spotted that would have otherwise gone unnoticed.

While it may seem creepy to think someone can tell your mood based on smartphone data, such technologies can help people when they are in a vulnerable place and may be prone to depression, such as after a job loss or after giving birth. These technologies take some of the subjectivity out of mental assessments, giving us real measurements. They could also help detect mental illness in loved ones. In the past decade, we've suffered a blight of unfortunate gun violence at the hands of individuals who were mentally unstable. How many lives could have been saved had there been interventions before those fateful days? And I'm not just referring to the mass killings that get widespread media attention—the well-known images we can recall from coverage at Newtown, Aurora, Charleston, and Virginia Tech. Since 2006, more than two hundred mass killings have occurred in the United States; they happen on average every two weeks.[6]

Mass killings, defined as four or more victims, take place far more often than the government reports, and the circumstances of those killings are far more predictable than you may think. The majority of cases are the result of breakups, estrangements, and family arguments, and often they involve a failed safety net. So picture a cell phone app that can provide that safety net. Once you've flagged the people you've designated in your safety net, the phone can send a message to them that something is wrong when it detects such a scenario, thereby providing a chance to prevent a tragedy. Exactly how these devices could be best used is still being studied, but they offer hope that maybe we can avert some of these horrible events in the future.

You're Part of the Cure with Big Data

The power of Big Data cannot be overstated. In 2013, a French study of nearly half a million people found that those who postpone retirement have less risk of developing Alzheimer's disease and other forms of dementia.[7] In fact, for each additional year of work, the risk of developing dementia is reduced by 3.2 percent. Not only does employment keep people physically active, but those people also stay more socially connected and mentally challenged. They are more likely to be confronted with new things to learn, which demands more focus and attention in the brain—all good things in terms of preventing mental decline.

That same year, another study found that living near an airport increases the risk for cardiovascular disease.[8] Among the 3.6 million people residing near Heathrow Airport in London, where this study was conducted by analyzing data, people who lived in the noisiest areas had a heightened risk for stroke, coronary heart disease, cardiovascular disease, hospital admissions, and death. What's more, in a similar analysis of data collected on more than 6 million people on Medicare who lived in zip codes around eighty-nine North American airports, researchers discovered that people who lived near airports ranked among the top 10 percent in terms of noise exposure also had a significant increase in the risk of hospital admission for cardiovascular disease, even after adjusting for age, sex, race, zip code–level socioeconomic status and demographics, zip code–level air pollution, and roadway density.[9] In fact, they calculated that for older people living near airports, 2.3 percent of hospitalizations for cardiovascular disease could be attributed to aircraft noise!

These studies required researchers to dig into reams of data that were probably not very well organized. Now, what if our hypothetical database of the future, which is filled with people's information regarding their basic habits and physiology, could ferret out all of these risk factors and important details seamlessly and effortlessly? Imagine the kinds of health management tools we could build around knowing, for example, the potential risks associated with your zip code or choice to retire at age seventy.

For another example, let's say you're an avid runner in your forties who has had a nagging pain in your hip. After a few referrals to doctors to help diagnose the problem, it's determined that you've got arthritis blooming in your hip (the same kind that your mother of seventy-five years young has, too; she's already had one replaced). You're told to stop running forever and take up a new, nonimpact sport. This isn't acceptable, and you vow to find an alternative solution. That solution could very well reside in this database, where scores of people like you in age, athletic proclivities, and diagnosis have insights about how to address your problem and totally overcome it without saying good-bye to the sport. Wouldn't that be life changing? Wouldn't the ability to mine other people's data be worth the risk of entering your own information into that database? I think so.

The point is your health information is part of the solution. You're not giving *up* anything—you're *giving*. And you're going to get back. You want to benefit from every patient who has gone before you. You might even find out that for your particular condition and your personal data, you don't need to be formally treated at all. Some diseases don't need traditional medicine, and some should probably be treated differently than they are today. Many cancers, such as low-grade prostate cancer, differentiated thyroid cancers, and some breast tumors, don't need treatment because their natural history is such that they won't harm you. But in our one-size-fits-all world, they are treated like any cancer, with aggressive treatments that entail side effects. We're all told to get a colonoscopy at age fifty, yet most people don't need it. If you have no polyps removed during the invasive procedure, then you didn't need it to begin with.

Similarly, asking a healthy man to undergo a prostate biopsy at age fifty just for screening purposes makes no sense. We need technology to determine who needs the tests. Over the next few years, I bet we'll move from recommending that everyone have a colonoscopy at age fifty to administering a blood test that can tell you whether you have a colon polyp. And if you do, then you can go on to have the procedure. The same is true with drugs like statins and aspirins; these medications have their place in medicine, but we are overusing them because we don't have a better way to determine exactly who should be taking them and when they should start. It's the medical equivalent of equipping everyone with an umbrella every day to cover the handful of people who truly need the umbrella when it rains in their city. Given our current lack of data, we just don't know which diseases need different treatments. Big Data will help us figure out that and so much more.

Here's one more case in point: Every year, approximately 300,000 Americans with appendicitis undergo emergency surgery under the assumption that if their appendix is not immediately removed, it will burst—with potentially fatal consequences. Your appendix is a little tubelike sac that's attached to the lower part of your large intestine on the right side. You can certainly live without it; it's likely a vestigial organ from our evolutionary past, though some say it could help reboot the digestive system with good bacteria after a diarrheal illness. But if you have to lose it due to infection, often from bad bacteria, it won't cause any known health problems.

Surgical treatment for appendicitis began in the 1880s. But is surgery always necessary? Today we know that the length of time that an appendix is inflamed isn't linked to the risk of it bursting. During the Cold War, when American sailors spent six months or more on nuclear submarines and were prohibited from surfacing, those who developed appendicitis didn't have the luxury of undergoing surgery. They were instead treated with antibiotics. And this course of therapy worked great overall; there were no deaths or complications reported. But this approach wasn't widely publicized. In 1961, during the height of the Cold War, Leonid Rogozov, a Russian doctor stationed in Antarctica, became desperate when his appendix became inflamed, so he cut it out himself. It would take another fifty-four years for us to realize that invasive surgery isn't always necessary. The self-surgery that saved Rogozov's life became big news in the Soviet press, and the doctor went on to specialize in surgery, dying in 2000 from lung cancer at the age of sixty-six.

In 2015, five small European studies involving about one thousand patients showed that antibiotics can cure some patients with appendicitis; roughly 70 percent of patients who took the antibiotics did not need surgery.[10] And those who wound up having an appendectomy after trying antibiotics first did not face any more complications than those who underwent surgery immediately. The opportunity to avoid more than two hundred thousand surgeries annually has been available since the dawn of antibiotics more than eighty years ago, but we didn't have the data to help us realize it. Now we do.

In the spring of 2015, a headline caught my attention that spotlights another angle to this data story. It read, "Like Sleeping Beauty, some research lies dormant for decades . . ."[11] A new study from the Indiana

University Bloomington School of Informatics and Computing's Center for Complex Networks and Systems Research attempted to answer the question of why some research papers and discoveries fade into obscurity for years, sometimes decades, and then suddenly the research explodes and finally has everyone's attention.

Surprisingly, the top journals for sleeping beauties are among the most prestigious: *Proceedings of the National Academy of Sciences* (in which this particular study was published), *Nature*, and *Science*. The fields with the highest rate of delayed acknowledgment included physics, chemistry, multidisciplinary science, mathematics, and general and internal medicine. Several papers in these categories experienced hibernation periods of more than seventy years. The "drowsiest sleeping beauty" in the study came from Karl Pearson, an influential statistician at the turn of the twentieth century. His paper, entitled "On Lines and Planes of Closest Fit to Systems of Points in Space," was published in 1901 in *Philosophical* magazine but did not "awaken" until 2002. Four of the top fifteen sleeping beauties identified by this latest study were published more than one hundred years ago! What the IU researchers determined is that a paper can be ahead of its time—unable to gain the attention of others given the prevailing assumptions and general philosophies of the day.

Findings like this would make anyone wonder what gems exist already in the literature to solve serious challenges today in health care. Although it was previously thought that long-dormant studies are few and far between, this new study shows that that clearly isn't the case. We must figure out the trigger mechanisms for awakening these sleeping beauties.

Trend Spotting

Collecting and recording health data goes far back in history. It's actually as old as writing itself, but it would take centuries for such data to be gathered and documented in a way that would be useful to the public. It would take, in fact, until the Middle Ages for the world to have its first public health data set, thanks in part to the spread of the bubonic plague.

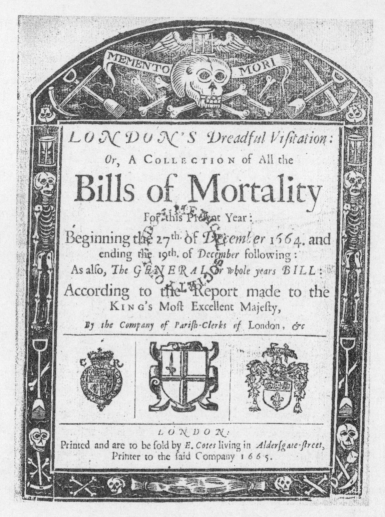

The title page for *Bills of Mortality* from 1664 and 1665.

In 1538, the English passed a law that required death certificates for burials. Apparently, the government was concerned that people were cheating on their taxes by pretending to be dead. Although the printing press had been invented nearly a century earlier, it wasn't until 1600 that someone thought of gathering all the death certificates and compiling them in order to see generally what was going on. Then the king would know who had died recently and would have a broad sense of his population's dynamics, for births were also listed. Eventually, this led to one-page weekly reports that documented who died and from what. These reports were called Bills of Mortality, and one particular set would go down in history as being among the most important texts in human history.

The Bills of Mortality is probably a literary collection you never studied in school.[12] It kept track of the rise and fall of the bubonic plague that struck England in 1664 and 1665. By most measures, it was the first record in the world of the spread of disease. Many of the recorded causes of death have odd-sounding names for us in modern times. Those who were charged with recording the deaths were not trained medical professionals, so they often fell short of knowing how to articulate the exact cause of death and would list peculiar or vague causes. Some deaths, for example, were listed as "griping in the guts," "grief," "suddenly," "frighted," and "stopping of the stomach." The recordings reveal that infant mortality rates were high. The children who died were usually categorized by their ages rather than listed according to the illnesses that might have killed them. Hence, infants younger than a month old were listed as "chrisomes" and babies who hadn't finished teething were listed as "teeth."

The Black Death peaked during the hot summer of 1665 in London. By mid-July, there were more than a thousand deaths a week, reported on handbills posted in public places to warn people that the plague was spreading. Many of the rich left the city, leaving the poor to die in droves. Shown on the following pages are three bills from that year, each of which lists the number of deaths in London for one week. The first one shows a week in February, during which one person died of plague while eighty-nine died of consumption (tuberculosis). By September, as seen in the second image, the plague killed 7,165 in one week. And by December, the third image, the numbers had declined, completing the epidemic curve of the year's outbreak.

This was the first time in human history that a pattern was reflected in the data; you could see the plague begin its march through the city

The Diseases and Casualties this Week.

Abortive	2	Imposthume	1
Aged	38	Infants	15
Apoplexie	1	Lethargy	1
Cancer	1	Overlaid	1
Canker	1	Kild 3, one at St. Margaret Westminster, and one in a Brewers Malt-mill, at St. Martin Vintery, and one by a fall from a Ladder at St. Giles in the Fields	3
Chilbed	6	Plague	1
Chrisoms	15	Rickets	6
Consumption	89	Rising of the Lights	6
Convulsion	43	Rupture	1
Cough	1	Scowring	3
Dropsie	44	Spotted Feaver	4
Drowned at Lambeth	3	Stilborn	11
Feaver	35	Stone	1
Flox and Small-pox	30	Stopping of the stomach	15
Flux	2	Suddenly	1
French-pox	3	Surfeit	6
Gowt	3	Teeth	22
Grief	1	Thrush	3
Griping in the Guts	14	Timpany	2
Jaundies	1	Tissick	16
		Ulcer	3
		Winde	3
		Wormes	4

Christned { Males — 113, Females - 111, In all — 224 } Buried { Males — 239, Females - 223, In all — 462 } Plague — 1

Increased in the Burials this Week —————— 69

Parishes cleat of the Plague ——— 129   Parishes Infected ——— 1

The Assize of Bread set forth by Order of the Lord Maior and Court of Aldermen, A penny Wheaten Loaf to contain Eleven Ounces and a half, and three half-penny White Loaves the like weight.

The list of deaths for the week of February 7 to 14, 1665, showing just one plague death at the beginning of the Black Death.

starting in the late spring, then kill scores of people during those warm summer months, and finally peter out again in the fall. In the words of my friend Jay Walker—who owns a leather-bound and vellum-paged volume of the original bills (the pages shown are from his volume) in his expansive, private Walker Library of the History of Human Imagination

The Difeafes and Cafualties this Week.

		Impofthume	11
		Infants	16
		Killed by a fall from the Belfrey at Alhallows the Great	1
		Kingfevil	2
		Lethargy	1
		Palfie	1
		Plague	7165
Abortive	5	Rickets	17
Aged	43	Rifing of the Lights	11
Ague	2	Scowring	5
Apoplexie	1	Scurvy	2
Bleeding	2	Spleen	1
Burnt in his Bed by a Candle at St. Giles Cripplegate	1	Spotted Feaver	101
		Stilborn	17
Canker	1	Stone	2
Childbed	42	Stopping of the ftomach	9
Chrifomes	18	Strangury	1
Confumption	134	Suddenly	1
Convulfion	64	Surfeit	49
Cough	2	Teeth	121
Dropfie	33	Thrufh	5
Feaver	309	Timpany	1
Flox and Small-pox	5	Tiffick	11
Frighted	3	Vomiting	3
Gowt	1	Winde	3
Grief	3	Wormes	15
Griping in the Guts	51		
Jaundies	5		

Chriftned { Males — 95, Females — 81, In all — 176 } Buried { Males — 4095, Females — 4202, In all — 8297 } Plague — 7165

Increafed in the Burials this Week — 607
Parifhes clear of the Plague — 4   Parifhes Infected — 126

The Affize of Bread fet forth by Order of the Lord Maior and Court of Aldermen, A penny Wheaten Loaf to contain Nine Ounces and a half, and three half-penny White Loaves the like weight.

The list of deaths for the week of September 12 to 19, 1665, showing 7,165 plague deaths during the peak of the Black Death.

in Connecticut—"The good Lord isn't plucking people out at random; he's plucking people out on a plague curve." From the Bills of Mortality came the notion that you can predict plague. Matters of public health can be charted, quantified, mathematized, and predicted.

We owe the actual organization and analysis of London's vital sta-

The list of deaths for the week of December 5 to 12, 1665, showing 243 plague deaths during the decline of the Black Death.

tistics to a man named John Graunt. Many historians credit him with establishing the science of demography, the statistical study of human populations. In honor of his work, Graunt was named a charter member of England's Royal Society, which is composed of prominent scientists.

Today we are all aware of patterns in the spread of illnesses, especially the infectious ones. Unlike the plague, which is carried by fleas that live as parasites on rats (hence the summer peak when the fleas proliferate in the warmth), the influenza virus peaks in the winter, when people are living mostly indoors in closer proximity. But we can misinterpret our data despite much better technology than that of the Middle Ages. You see, data without context is meaningless. A few years ago, when Google tried to predict the spread of flu using its search engine, it got it wrong. By comparing traditional surveillance data with Google Flu Trends' results, which were derived from the number of flu-related internet searches, it was shown that Google had drastically overestimated peak flu levels, and did so three years in a row.[13] This was yet another reminder that while high-tech flu-tracking techniques based on mining of web data and on social media can be useful, they will complement traditional epidemiological surveillance networks until the technology can fully substitute them.

The problem that Google faced was a basic foible of artificial intelligence: computers and search engines are deftly clever at tracing what people are searching for ("fever," "flu," "sore throat," "chills, fever, body aches," "symptoms of flu"), but they can't tell if those people are actually sick. So healthy people in Seattle, for example, searching for facts about the flu and its symptoms—maybe a class of children searching for information for a school report, or someone who just heard a news report about the flu in the local media—can skew the search engine's tracking algorithm. They are creating the wrong context for Google to do its thing. They are, put simply, the wrong messenger—unknowingly sabotaging the system because Google tags them as potential flu patients when in fact they are not and might never be that year.

Misleading messages like this are everywhere today, and the volume of health information and even health opinions out there makes it hard to know whom and what to trust. It also makes the discovery of your own context to inform your decisions all the more challenging. I'll be helping you define your current context. But first, we must address what it means to move at the speed of health.

CHAPTER 4

The Dawn of Precision Medicine

How to Manage Its Power and Perils

*I personally think we are just not smart enough—and won't be
for a very long time—to feel comfortable about the consequences
of changing heredity, even in a single individual.*[1]

—David Baltimore, former president of Caltech and
1975 Nobel laureate in Physiology or Medicine

N o sooner did the world realize that we could begin to edit any
gene in the human genome than a group of scientists, including
those who pioneered the technology, called for a worldwide morato-
rium on using the new technique. They argued, in an article for *Science*
in 2015, that this would give us all time to understand the issues surrounding this breakthrough method fully.[2] David Baltimore was one of
the paper's authors concerned about the dangers of altering the human
genome, claiming that we're not "smart enough" to understand the potential consequences of tinkering with the very makeup of our species
and artificially reshaping human genetics.

When you make changes to the genome, it means you modify human
sperm, eggs, or embryos in a way that will be permanent throughout the
life of that individual and then will be passed on to future generations

of biological children and their descendants. Until now, these worries were theoretical. Today, however, we are living in a brave new reality. And the future of medicine—and of you and me—rests on figuring out which technologies we should make universally accessible and which we would do well to safeguard from widespread use. This safeguarding is not easy; the warning from David Baltimore's group came days after a group of Chinese scientists reported that they were already editing the genomes of human embryos.

The fact that there's no reliable governance over technologies as important as DNA screening and DNA editing is emblematic of the fact that most people are living purely in reactive mode when it comes to their health, and not in preventive mode. This is a huge problem in the modern age, when a person can go from Singapore to San Francisco in a day. Epidemics such as SARS (severe acute respiratory syndrome), avian flu, Ebola, or West Nile virus, to name a few in recent memory, can spread faster than ever before. We are poorly coordinated to handle a real and sudden catastrophe if one hit. We fail to think toward the future and make reasonable predictions based on known parameters.

In the past few years, there's been a surge in parasitic brain-eating amoebas infecting people who swim in warm lake waters. Two children died in 2012 after swimming in Minnesota's Lily Lake, near the Twin Cities, and one California woman succumbed to a fatal brain infection caused by the parasite in 2015. This particular type of amoeba can only thrive in warm conditions, and is typically found in Texas and Florida. But given the warming trends in recent years, the waters have changed—and so have their inhabitants. As a society, we need to be better at predicting such shifts so we can act quickly when unfamiliar foes emerge. The Department of Homeland Security was founded quickly after the September 11, 2001, attacks to help keep us one step ahead of the terrorists. It's time we established a Department of Homeland Health, whose sole purpose is to predict and prepare for all the biological threats out there—many of which are currently not within the purview of the Department of Health and Human Services or the Centers for Disease Control and Prevention.

Conversations about how to govern health in the future must happen now, from establishing the ethics around gene editing to setting up more reliable strategies for predicting pandemics. Once we make those decisions, we might be able to help people like Sharon Bernardi and the seven children she lost, six of whom died within hours or days of birth and one who lived until he was twenty-one.

Three-Parent Babies

Sharon Bernardi wasn't unlike many young women hoping to become a mother and have a family.[3] But her first three pregnancies, all of which were uneventful, resulted in babies who died soon after they were born. It was discovered that their fragile little bodies mysteriously began to accumulate acid in their blood upon their birth that caused their swift departure. At the time, no one could explain it. This was when Sharon's mother shared that she, too, had lost three babies to stillbirth before Sharon, her only surviving child.

It took Sharon and her husband a long time to get over the loss of their first baby, which came as a shock given how good she'd felt during the pregnancy and how normal the birth was. But then it happened again and again. Every time Sharon got pregnant, she prayed the horror wouldn't repeat. Although her doctors began to have a feeling that the deaths were connected somehow, they couldn't make sense of it. An early genetic investigation led nowhere. They did, however, note that members of Sharon's extended family had also lost children—a breathtaking eight children in all beyond Sharon's. And then came Edward.

Edward was Sharon's fourth attempt to have a healthy biological child whom she wouldn't have to bury prematurely. This time the doctors took a more cautious, prepared approach to the delivery. Edward received drugs and blood transfusions for his first forty-eight hours after being born. This was to prevent the lactic acidosis—the blood poisoning—that had killed his siblings. And he survived. Five weeks later, Sharon and her husband, Neil, took Edward home to Sunderland in the United Kingdom for Christmas. He developed normally, reaching all his early milestones: he sat up, he crawled, and at fourteen months, he started to walk. Overall, he was a happy, active boy, but his mother did have to care for him a lot and he didn't seem as healthy as other kids his age did.

The signs of serious trouble started when Edward was about two. That's when he began to fall down repeatedly when trying to walk. And then he started having seizures, which helped doctors arrive at the root source of the problem with all of Sharon's children. In 1994, when Edward was four, doctors finally diagnosed him with Leigh's disease, a disorder that affects the central nervous system. It leads to a variety of challenges such as loss of head control and motor skills, learning difficulties, and impairment of breathing and kidney function. Most children don't live long with Leigh's disease, as it progresses rapidly. Doctors told Sharon that her son would probably not make it to kindergarten. She learned that Edward would have intervals of remission amid periods of illness that could happen suddenly. And his seizures were especially worrisome, for they could last for days, and doctors thought he'd die during one of these prolonged episodes.

Sharon and Neil continued to try for a healthy baby. But there'd be no such luck. She gave birth to three more children, but none lived beyond the age of two. After each death, Sharon and Neil comforted themselves by saying the death was "a one-off." Perhaps it's just human nature to think like that, especially when you're aching for a healthy child. But after their last child had a heart attack and died in 2000, they stopped pursuing another pregnancy. After all, they still had Edward, and he'd already lived long past what the doctors had predicted.

Edward was a lucky one who enjoyed life through his teenage years and into young adulthood. He then experienced a steady weakening of his condition until he died from a cardiac arrest in 2011 following a year of chronic pain and severe muscular spasms caused by the chaotic, incurable disorder in his brain. Drugs could not help him.

Although people have criticized Sharon and Neil's choices, accusing them of being selfish for wanting what they couldn't have—biological children—their story now stands front and center of a debate about

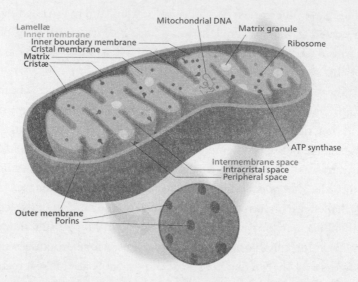

Lamellæ
Inner membrane
Inner boundary membrane
Cristal membrane
Matrix
Cristæ

Mitochondrial DNA
Matrix granule
Ribosome

ATP synthase
Intermembrane space
Intracristal space
Peripheral space

Outer membrane
Porins

The structure of the mitochondrion. These tiny "organelles" are the cell's energy packers—they are responsible for creating more than 90 percent of the energy needed by the body to sustain life and support growth. Damage to these vital compartments can cause an array of disorders, from those of the musculature to serious neurological conditions. Mitochondrial diseases inflict the most damage to cells of the brain, heart, liver, skeletal muscles, kidney, and the endocrine and respiratory systems. The mitochondria have their own DNA coding for 37 genes, containing approximately 16,600 base pairs.

what medicine can finally offer such couples: a disease-free child. But there's a catch: the child will have three parents—two mothers and a father—at least genetically speaking. For Sharon, it's not so much her own suffering that has convinced her of the need to develop genetic therapies that would allow mitochondrial defects to become a thing of the past, or at least be remedied. It's about the children's suffering. And this breathtaking technology is taking flight.

The mitochondria, sometimes referred to as the cells' internal power plants, are tiny structures within our cells that have their own DNA separate from the DNA in the nucleus of the cell. They contain anywhere from five to ten copies of their DNA, whereas the nucleus of the cell contains only two copies of its DNA. Mitochondria are found in all cells except red blood cells and generate energy in the form of a chemical called ATP (adenosine triphosphate). German doctor Carl Benda first identified them in 1897, noting that these particles looked like tiny threadlike grains. Hence the name *mitochondria*, derived from the Greek *mitos*, meaning "thread," and *chondrin*, meaning "grain."

In 1949 the mitochondria's role as cellular powerhouses was finally explained by two American scientists, Eugene Kennedy and Albert Lehninger. Basically, mitochondria conduct chemical reactions that convert certain molecules and nutrients into the energy that powers most cell functions. It helps to think of mitochondria as cellular batteries. The energy-rich ATP they produce can be delivered throughout the cell as needed in the presence of specific enzymes. The cells in your brain, muscles, heart, kidney, and liver contain thousands of mitochondria each. And in some cells, mitochondria comprise up to 40 percent of the material.

The current thinking is that our mitochondria were once free-living bacterial organisms that eventually became part of our own cells, providing the benefit of producing energy. As a result, each single mitochondrion contains its own genome, but it doesn't have all the genes it needs to function independently (it contains just 37 genes as opposed to the approximately 20,000 to 25,000 protein-coding genes found in the nucleus of cells). Like bacterial DNA, the DNA of the mitochondria is arranged in a circle, quite unlike the genetic material found within the nucleus of the cell. Also unlike our nuclear genome, which includes chromosomes from both parents, all of a person's mitochondria originate from the thousands contained in the mother's egg. In other words, it's inherited solely from the female lineage. During reproduction, while the nuclear DNA of the sperm joins with that of the egg, the male's mitochondria are excluded. This is the basis by which scientists use the term "Mitochondrial Eve," referring to the first human mother from whom all humans have derived some of their mitochondrial DNA. She is thought to have lived some 170,000 years ago in East Africa when we *Homo sapiens* were evolving as a species separate from other hominids.

The mitochondrial genome is not nearly as stable as the nuclear genome. For reasons that science is still trying to figure out, mitochondrial

genes accrue random mutations about 1,000 times faster than nuclear
DNA. As many as 1 in 5,000 children are born with diseases caused by
these mutations, which affect cells that demand lots of energy, such as
those in the brain and muscles. The proportion of diseased mitochondria that a mother passes on to her children determines the severity of
the conditions.

Mitochondrial diseases include neurological, muscular, and metabolic disorders; diseases as diverse as diabetes, some forms of autism,
Parkinson's, Alzheimer's, and even cancer have all been linked to mitochondrial problems.[4] So the question becomes: can we eradicate these
mitochondrial defects? Enter someone like Douglass Turnbull.

Correcting Blips in DNA[5]

Douglass Turnbull is a professor of neurology at Newcastle University in
the United Kingdom, where he conducts research and is director of the
Wellcome Trust Centre for Mitochondrial Research. After years of watching patients with untreatable and sometimes fatal mitochondrial diseases,
including Sharon Bernardi and her children, he vowed to find a way to
prevent mitochondrial disorders like Leigh's disease from being passed
on. He first got interested in mitochondrial diseases nearly forty years ago
when he was working in a neurology ward and came across a member
of the Royal Air Force who complained of severe muscle weakness on
training runs. Although Turnbull was wrong to suspect a mitochondrial
disease in this particular man, the subject nonetheless intrigued him.
He then went on to earn an MD and a PhD, the latter of which focused
on understanding the molecular mechanisms in mitochondrial disease.
He's devoted his career to understanding how these vital little structures,
which have a life of their own inside cells, malfunction.

It was Turnbull who found out that Sharon carried mutant mitochondria when he met her in the mid-1990s and had her undergo a
muscle biopsy. He was surprised that Sharon looked so well, but he
wasn't surprised to hear that many of her family members had suffered
major health challenges. Sharon herself began to have health issues at

the age of thirty-five. Her mother started to experience heart difficulties in her mid-fifties. Turnbull was determined to prevent kids from inheriting bad mitochondria.

Dr. Turnbull wasn't the first to think about wiping out mutant mitochondria. In the 1980s, embryologists working with mice began exploring possible techniques for doing so. The procedure they discovered, sometimes called three-person in vitro fertilization (IVF), involves transferring the genetic material from the cell's nucleus (the 23 pairs of chromosomes) from the egg of a woman with mutant mitochondria into another woman's healthy egg. This eliminates defective mitochondria while preserving the biological mother's chromosomal DNA. The procedure can be done in a couple of ways (see page 110).

Turnbull and other scientists have experimented with this technique in monkeys, mice, and human egg cells in culture. In 2009, at the Oregon Health & Science University in Beaverton, stem-cell and reproductive biologist Shoukhrat Mitalipov and his colleagues announced the birth of two healthy rhesus macaques whose nuclei and mitochondria had come from different egg cells. At their fifth birthdays, they were still as healthy as could be. Mitalipov and his team have also demonstrated their procedure in human eggs: they created embryos that developed into formed blastocysts—cellular masses of between 50 and 200 stem cells that have the potential to develop into any of the body's different tissues. These blastocysts could be transplanted into a woman's uterus. Now the team is eager to do just that and test their method out in humans.

The procedures do have their critics, and for obvious reasons. Could these techniques have unintended consequences? For example, could they trigger small changes at the molecular or genetic level that impact development or trigger health problems later in life? This is possible, if there are unforeseen incompatibilities between the mitochondrial and nuclear genomes in individuals conceived using such techniques. For the mitochondria to function properly, the mitochondrial genes need to be compatible with the individual's own DNA. Genetic variations in both structures probably evolved together. Several studies have shown that replacing the mitochondria in mice, fruit flies, and other organisms

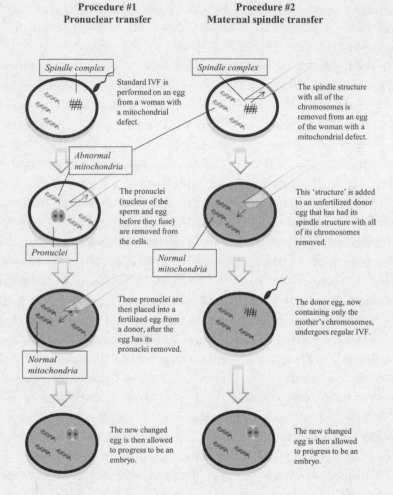

Procedure #1
Pronuclear transfer

Procedure #2
Maternal spindle transfer

Spindle complex

Spindle complex

Standard IVF is performed on an egg from a woman with a mitochondrial defect.

The spindle structure with all of the chromosomes is removed from an egg of the woman with a mitochondrial defect.

Abnormal mitochondria

The pronuclei (nucleus of the sperm and egg before they fuse) are removed from the cells.

This 'structure' is added to an unfertilized donor egg that has had its spindle structure with all of its chromosomes removed.

Pronuclei

Normal mitochondria

These pronuclei are then placed into a fertilized egg from a donor, after the egg has its pronuclei removed.

The donor egg, now containing only the mother's chromosomes, undergoes regular IVF.

Normal mitochondria

The new changed egg is then allowed to progress to be an embryo.

The new changed egg is then allowed to progress to be an embryo.

This diagram demonstrates the two procedures capable of fusing a diseased egg with a healthy one to prevent rare but devastating mitochondrial diseases.

can sometimes result in issues with breathing, fertility, and cognition. So how can we be sure the technique is safe for all involved? And does this technology place us on the top of a steep slope down which we can easily slide to creating "designer babies"?

Compared to what's going on in Britain, we're far behind in talking about these developments and how to regulate them nationally and globally. And yet the technology is already at our fingertips. It's been here for much longer than anyone probably realizes, and even the FDA has had to play catch-up. Since 2001, the FDA has required researchers to gain permission for mitochondrial transfers. This came after a fertility clinic in New Jersey performed numerous procedures that transferred small amounts of cytoplasm—and some of their mitochondria—between human eggs to help women conceive. It happened in the mid-1990s, the same time Sharon Bernardi was grieving her deceased children, and her doctors were finally beginning to understand their demise. A fertility specialist named Jacques Cohen, then at Saint Barnabas Medical Center in Livingston, New Jersey, conducted an experiment that achieved mitochondrial replacement. At the time he was trying to treat a handful of women who were unable to conceive on their own. These women had eggs that were still young enough to produce healthy children, but the cytoplasm around their nuclei didn't look good.

The cytoplasm of a cell is a thick, gel-like solution that encompasses the area around the nucleus and is enclosed by the cell membrane. It's about 80 percent water and includes all of the material inside the cell and outside the nucleus, including the mitochondria. In Cohen's infertile patients, the cytoplasm appeared fragmented and filled with debris, which led him to wonder what would happen if he added some cytoplasm from another woman's healthy egg, thereby "rejuvenating" the egg.

After his first attempt in mice worked, he tested the technique in humans in 1997, rejuvenating the eggs of 33 infertile women with a careful squirt of cytoplasm from another woman's egg. Nine months later, 17 babies were born as a result. Cohen knew that the transplanted cytoplasm likely contained the "cellular battery packs known as mitochondria" that would support embryo development. But he probably had no idea at the time that his team was actually changing each egg's mitochondrial DNA, pioneering a way to tinker with a human's genetic inheritance—and creating the world's first genetically modified humans. In 2001, tests emerged that confirmed that at least two babies had mitochondria from two sources: the cytoplasm donor and their own biological mother.

What happened—and what *will* happen—to these children? We don't know all the health implications. Studies in mice suggest that such mixed mitochondria can have unintended consequences. In mice, at least, it's been documented that they can become hypertensive and obese in middle age, and have impaired cognition. Among Cohen's new mothers, one of the babies born developed an autism spectrum disorder, and two of the fetuses, one of which was miscarried and the other aborted, had a serious genetic defect known as Turner's syndrome. Whether or not these defects were a direct result of the procedure is yet to be known. The team stopped performing the procedure in 2001, when the FDA cracked down, saying that more research was required before it could be applied for human use.

These 17 children are now teenagers, and nobody has formally followed up with them. Cohen is currently the lab director of Reprogenetics, a preimplantation genetic diagnostics company in Livingston, and he's on a hunt to see what happened to these children, if they are willing to be revealed and undergo further testing. He and his team hope their findings can further move the needle in this area of medicine and push the debate forward for the benefit of all of us.

The idea that we can edit our genes and even change the entire human genome of future generations might make Darwin shift in his grave, for he's the one who suggested that nature selects the best genes to live on and procreate, that nature—not human engineering—should be the ultimate judge. I sometimes wonder what he would think about the value of DNA sequencing when it can't tell the whole story or, worse, leads to unintended consequences such as unnecessary surgery or treatment that's costly and painful.

Art and Science Will Still Define Precision Medicine

We should remember that precision medicine is a double-edged sword. While it can open the door to new and better ways to take care of ourselves, it's not nearly as "precise" as most people think.

Let me start with a fictional character whose story mirrors what can happen in real life. We'll call him Larry. He's in his mid-thirties, which some say is the prime of life. He shouldn't be diagnosed with a rare, inoperable tumor. But he does indeed get such a grave diagnosis, and despite the best that conventional cancer medicine can offer him, the disease progresses rapidly. He finalizes plans for his family's future, including his two young children, and prepares to enter hospice care, thinking that he's got days, maybe weeks, to live. And that's when he consents to having his tumor sequenced, a strategy he hadn't contemplated before. It reveals a mutation in a gene that appears to be driving the growth of the cancer. Better yet, it shows that his cancer could be targeted with a particular drug, but one not normally used for his type of cancer. With nothing to lose, he starts taking the pills. And the tumor shrinks. Months later, he is still alive and no longer a candidate for hospice care.

Some would say that story exemplifies personalized or precision medicine—the medicine of the future, in which we will tailor treatments to a person's unique physiology and health condition. But this approach is far from new. From Charaka, the father of ancient Indian practices (Ayurveda) to Hippocrates, the first father of modern medicine, many doctors throughout history have practiced the personalized approach to some degree using available technology for treating a disease. Today, however, personalized medicine is much more precise from a molecular standpoint. It focuses chiefly on DNA and how single-nucleotide polymorphisms (SNPs) and environmental factors influence an individual's biology and risk for disease. SNPs are variations in DNA sequences that are thought to provide the genetic markers for our response to disease and drugs. For example, a variation on a particular gene may indicate a predisposition for high cholesterol. Other variations may provide a marker for celiac disease or indicate a higher risk for Alzheimer's.

It's important to realize that these DNA differences do not *cause* the disease, but they are a marker of the relative risk of the disease. Since the completion of the Human Genome Project in 2003, hundreds of published, peer-reviewed studies have described the associations between SNPs and specific diseases, traits, and conditions. As you can imagine, these studies have opened the door for the personal genomics industry by providing a platform by which DNA, obtained through a simple saliva sample or tube of blood, can reveal your individual genetic map. It's also the platform behind sequencing tumors and understanding their characteristics within the context of the body's DNA.

Personalized medicine has its limitations amid its promises. At the end of January 2015, President Obama presented his new Precision Medicine Initiative during the State of the Union address. He said the goal is "delivering the right treatment at the right time, every time, to the right person." To fund the initiative, Obama asked Congress for $215 million, more than half of which would help the National Institutes of Health (NIH) develop "one of the largest research populations ever assembled," a group of at least 1 million volunteers who would share genomic data, lifestyle information, and biological samples. This data would further be linked to their electronic health records. The National Cancer Institute (NCI) would receive another $70 million to support efforts to identify genes that spur malignant tumor development, an endeavor first proposed by the NIH's director, Dr. Francis Collins, more than a decade before.

While this project is honorable, it can ignore the bigger picture and downplay basic preventive measures such as diet and exercise that aren't as sexy as taking pills to tinker with genes. And therein lies the main challenge of precision medicine: it implies that if you know your genome, you can fit treatments to it. But that's a reductionist view—it's looking at just one chunk of the information, much of which could actually be useless in terms of knowing true risk factors and longevity. It also misses the value of prevention. For example, if we're going to prevent the 86 million adults who are currently prediabetic from being diagnosed with diabetes in the next decade, it's not going to come from sequencing DNA and prescribing molecular therapies. It'll happen through old-fashioned diet and exercise.

Cardiologist Eric Topol, director of the Scripps Translational Science Institute, stated it perfectly in an article for the *Journal of the American Medical Association*: "If you really want to change medicine, you have to have all the information on the individual. That includes their environment, the bacteria in their gut, and other distinguishing characteristics."[6] And he's right. Precision medicine's greatest prospects, at least in the short term, lie in the development of cancer therapeutics and pharmacogenomics, the customization of drugs and dosages to fit a person's genetic profile.

The power and utility of pharmacogenomics is exemplified by a 2015 study that found that children with acute lymphoblastic leukemia (a type of cancer in which the bone marrow makes too many immature white blood cells) and a particular genetic variation in their DNA were at greater risk for experiencing severe nerve damage when treated with the drug vincristine.[7] Such a finding can inform safer dosing of this widely used anticancer drug. Thus far, labels on more than 150 medications contain pharmacogenomic information, although genetic testing before use isn't necessarily recommended.

The allure of drugs that target mutant DNA and more or less play with our internal switches does indeed sound appealing, as well as exciting. But along with the lack of context this approach gives you, there is a big hurdle to clear, which few people like to talk about: the pricing. During his presentation at the White House as chronicled in the *JAMA* article, Obama showcased William Elder Jr., a twenty-seven-year-old man who was born with the inherited DNA for cystic fibrosis, a disorder triggered by a rare genetic defect that causes severe damage to the lungs and digestive system and can be life threatening. William had already been living with symptoms of the condition for twenty years when Obama introduced him. He was in medical school and had every intention to live to see his grandchildren. In 2012, William started a new drug designed to target the specific defect that causes cystic fibrosis and the effects were almost immediate: his breathing improved within hours.

But these breaths do come with a hefty price. The drug he takes, ivacaftor (Kalydeco), costs $300,000 annually. And it's not even a universal cure for the disease. Kalydeco is approved for treating patients with any of ten specific mutations in the cystic fibrosis gene. Patients like William, who have one of those ten mutations, represent fewer than 10 percent of the thirty thousand or so individuals with the disease in the United States, according to the Cystic Fibrosis Foundation. Vertex, the company that manufactures Kalydeco, plans to market the medication alongside another experimental drug that treats the cystic fibrosis genetic defect associated with half of the cases in the United States. The company is also investigating the drug combination in people with another type of mutation that causes cystic fibrosis.

Is the $300,000 price tag fair? As I mentioned, I routinely witness new anticancer drugs on the market that come with exorbitant price tags and may buy only a few more days or weeks of life. In the future, we will have to figure out the real value of these drugs and how to pay for them. Cost should be driven by benefit, with what's called value-based pricing. If you have a drug that buys five to ten more years of life, it should cost more than the drug that provides minimal benefits. The current model is untenable if drug companies can charge whatever they want—especially given the fact that many of these new drugs work best in combination with other drugs, multiplying the costs by two or three.

The irony of this is that technology costs have come down considerably in the past decade, but not the cost of drugs. And that will have to change if we're going to enjoy this brave new world of medicine. The predatory practice of pricing as high as possible for a new drug is inappropriate, and I am simply calling for an orderly system with guidelines. We have to provide incentives for biotechnology and pharmaceutical companies to make progress and take risks. But just because their patents give them a temporary monopoly on the market, that doesn't mean prices should reflect that. Change will happen faster once more doctors and hospitals stand up to the pharmaceutical industry and compel it to establish a more rational and transparent approach to drug pricing. Memorial Sloan Kettering Cancer Center in New York City, for example, has invented an interactive calculator (www.drugabacus.org) that compares the current cost of more than fifty cancer drugs with what the prices would be if those drugs were tied to factors such as how much they extend the life of patients and the side effects those patients endure. It's a smart idea: fix prices to real values, which for patients are quality and length of life. Memorial's project has shown that in many cases, the calculator computes a price that is lower than the drug's market price. And of course, this includes the cost of developing the drug.

Although people like to lament the power of Big Pharma, doctors and hospitals can also score some victories. In 2012, Memorial Sloan Kettering decided not to give its patients with colorectal cancer the drug aflibercept (Zaltrap), a new product made by Sanofi, the world's fifth-largest pharmaceutical company. Originally, the drug cost $11,000 per month, and the doctors didn't think the effects of the drug justified such a high price tag. So they banded together, wrote a newspaper editorial laying out their decision, and Sanofi relented, cutting the price by 50 percent for oncologists like me in the United States.

Even with lowered price tags, many in the medical community question whether focusing on the genetic underpinnings of disease is the most cost-effective approach when it comes to improving health. And even I can sympathize with this concern. Precisely because I cofounded a company that performed genetic screening, I can say that genes don't tell the whole story. In lectures, I like to use the following analogy: you can take a car apart and examine all of its pieces, but that won't tell you how long it will take to drive that car from point A to B. In addition to the car parts, you have to consider how those parts work together in a complex system. You have to consider the quality of the oil and gasoline, as well as the environment in which the car is moving. And you have to think about all the other variables that help determine the car's functionality, from weather and road conditions to the driver's competency, the traffic, and the path taken.

Obama's Precision Medicine Initiative isn't the first to create a database to collect and mine health information with a focus on genomics. The NIH has already launched three trials to study patients' cancers for genetic abnormalities. Then patients can be enrolled into an appropriate clinical trial of an investigational drug that might hit the specific molecular blips, or "on" switches, driving their cancer. One of these trials is the NCI-MATCH (Molecular Analysis for Therapy Choice) trial, which is accepting adults with cancers that have stopped responding to traditional treatment. Pediatric MATCH is the one for children.

And the third trial is the Lung Cancer Master Protocol for Squamous Cell Carcinoma, or Lung-MAP—a collaborative effort between private and public sectors that implements a similar molecular approach for people with squamous cell lung cancer, which currently lacks effective treatments other than surgery. The Dana-Farber Cancer Institute also launched its Profile program in September 2011. It's the first hospital in the United States to provide tumor genotyping to all patients with cancer. The goal is to create a large-scale study similar to the famous Framingham Heart Study, which laid the foundation for a great number of cardiovascular disease studies over the past half-century. These large-scale studies should help us learn the answers to questions like: Do cancer patients with a variation in gene X live longer or shorter? In the words of the NIH's Francis Collins, eventually the plan is to "generate the knowledge base necessary to move precision medicine into virtually all areas of health and disease."[8]

One thing to keep in mind is that precision medicine, no matter how technical it gets and useful it becomes across all fields of medicine, will always entail a little bit of art and science. Just as you can't buy devices and fully take care of yourself based on those alone, you can't rely on genomics to understand fully your body and how to treat it. DNA must be looked upon in the context of other things in your life. Take, for instance, the woman I mentioned earlier who was told a few years back she has a very high likelihood of developing Alzheimer's disease due to a gene variant, but several years later, she is told that she also has a protective gene that renders her risk as average. Or consider the woman who is informed she has an alteration in the BRCA1 gene that dramatically raises her risk of breast cancer. While she is considering having her breasts removed, a second opinion at a major cancer center tells her that the alteration she has in BRCA1 doesn't raise her risk for breast cancer at all. Her alteration is a variant that has no increased risk. All of these are true stories of patients I have worked with, and they highlight the complexity and the evolving nature of modern medicine. Despite the progress and promise in the study of DNA, it's just a small fraction of the total amount of information contained in your body.

Your Genes Have Friendly Neighbors

Earlier I noted how mitochondria, the energy source in our cells, were once free-living bacteria that somehow ended up getting incorporated into our physiology to power life. It turns out that we owe our life—and health—to more microbes than we ever imagined before. In fact, one can argue we owe our life more to these microbes than to our own DNA from a numbers standpoint: they outnumber our own cells by a factor of about 10 and include more than eight million genes. That amounts to more than 300 times the number of genes we contain in our own DNA. Luckily, our cells are much larger, so the microbes don't outweigh us 10 to 1. These microbes are found everywhere, inside and out. They cloak our mouth, nose, ears, intestines, genitalia, and skin. Scientists have so far identified some ten thousand species of microbes, including many that have never been documented before, but that number of species will probably climb and could approach thirty-five thousand. New technologies are emerging to help us identify all species, many of which cannot be cultured traditionally in a laboratory and demand high tech DNA sequencing to identify.

Most of these organisms make their home within our digestive tract, and while they include fungi and viruses, the bacterial species have starring roles in supporting our health. And we interact not only with these microbial organisms but also with their genetic material. The two million unique bacterial genes found in each human microbiome can make the 20,000 to 25,000 protein-coding genes in our cells seem almost negligible by comparison. Indeed, we are more microbial than human.

Even our own DNA has codes of viral origin. Throughout our evolution, viruses have inserted themselves into the human genome, and some could be responsible for our illnesses. Recent studies, for example, suggest that the deadly muscle degenerative disease amyotrophic lateral sclerosis (ALS), also known as Lou Gehrig's disease, could be associated with remnants of an ancient virus that entered our genome thousands of years ago. Although this research is just beginning, and a lot more needs to be understood—including environmental factors in the expression of genes that lead to the disease—the takeaway is that we're not just made up of human cells. We are an intricate web of microbial components that have a say in our lifelong biology.

As I mentioned earlier, the microbiome is our term for the complex microbial world that thrives outside of our own cells, but still within us (*micro* for "small" or "microscopic," and *biome* referring to a naturally occurring community of flora occupying a large habitat—in this case, the human body). Although the human genome is almost the same in every individual, give or take the genes that encode things like certain physical characteristics, risk factors for disease, and blood type, even identical twins can have hugely different gut profiles. The state of the microbiome is turning out to be so key to human health that it may actually be considered an organ in and of itself. And how we feel, both emotionally and physically, may hinge on the state of our microbiome. The NIH Human Microbiome Project started in 2008 as an extension of the Human Genome Project to catalog these microorganisms living in our body, and our appreciation for the influence of such organisms has grown rapidly with each passing year.[9]

Our growing knowledge about the microbiome comes from studying mice that have been altered so that they do not have any gut bacteria. This allows scientists to study the effects of missing microbes, or to expose the "germ-free" mice to various strains of bacteria and record changes in behavior. Germ-free lab rats have been shown, for example, to exhibit severe anxiety or have chronic gut and general inflammation, the latter of which is a huge risk factor for virtually every disease.[10] The studies on the impact artificial sweeteners can have on the microbiome, for instance, are among the many finally exposing the power these microbes can have in our own physiology and what can happen when their healthy balance is disrupted or otherwise compromised. Scientists have also documented a "diabetes fingerprint," a specific array of gut bacteria that correlates with the disease. Researchers can now manipulate gut bacteria in animal models, resulting in better blood sugar control and insulin sensitivity (important for controlling and even reversing type 2 diabetes). With more than 29 million Americans suffering from diabetes, this finding provides an incredible opportunity for both preventing and treating the disease, as well as addressing its complications, which include serious neurological conditions such as nerve damage, blindness, and dementia. About half of all Americans are affected by diabetes: they either have the metabolic disorder or are prediabetic.

In 2015, for another example, the journal *Nature* reported on the deleterious effects dietary emulsifiers have on the microbiome, at least in mice.[11] Emulsifiers are molecules that act as blending agents in food products that contain otherwise unmixable ingredients such as oil and water. They are ubiquitous in processed foods, including ice cream, salad dressing, and cream cheese. Look for names like carrageenan, lecithin, polysorbate 80, polyglycerols, guar gum, locust bean gum, carboxymethylcellulose, and xanthan gum in the packages you buy. Lecithin is actually nature's emulsifier; it's found in egg yolks and soy and is responsible for giving mayonnaise its creamy consistency.

Emulsifiers are also added to foods to extend their shelf life, improve texture, and keep ingredients from separating. In recent decades, there has been a significant increase in the number of people with metabolic syndrome and inflammatory bowel disease. Metabolic syndrome is not a disease in itself, but rather a group of risk factors that includes obesity, type 2 diabetes, and cardiovascular events such as heart attacks and strokes. Inflammatory bowel disease refers to inflammatory conditions of the colon and small intestine, such as ulcerative colitis and Crohn's disease. All of these illnesses are associated with changes in gut microbiota and, in turn, affect one's digestion.

Researchers have long been puzzled by the rising incidence of these illnesses, which can't be due to human genetics because that hasn't changed much in recent decades. This conundrum is what inspired Andrew Gewirtz, a biology professor at Georgia State University, to look for external environmental factors contributing to the increase. He and his colleagues used two groups of mice. One group had abnormal digestive systems that were predisposed to colitis, or inflammation of the colon. The other group had healthy digestive systems. When emulsifiers were given to the predisposed mice through water and food, the mice developed chronic colitis. The healthy mice developed low-grade intestinal inflammation and a metabolic disorder that caused them to eat more, becoming obese, hyperglycemic, and resistant to insulin.

Emulsifiers appear to disrupt the mucous layer that protects the intestinal tract, allowing for the movement of bacteria and increased inflammation as the body reacts to the bacteria being in the wrong place. The inflammatory response, in turn, interferes with satiety, or knowing instinctively when one has eaten enough. This, they theorize, caused the mice in the study to overeat and get fatter. Human studies are planned to see how much these emulsifiers are contributing to the obesity epidemic. Tests are also underway to determine if the natural emulsifier lecithin has the same effects as the chemical ones do.

Studies like that are just the beginning. Overall, what the latest science tells us is that our intestinal organisms participate in a wide variety of physiological actions, including immune system functioning, inflammation, hormonal functions, neurotransmitter and vitamin production, digestion and nutrient absorption, and detoxification. They help dictate whether we feel hungry or full, and how we utilize carbohydrates and fat. All of these processes factor into whether or not we develop conditions as diverse as diabetes, cancer, depression, or dementia. The microbiome affects our mood, libido, metabolism, immunity, and even our perception of the world and our thinking processes. Some of the latest science is showing that a disease long thought to be rooted in the brain—depression—may actually come from the gut, as well as depression's kissing cousins: chronic anxiety, insomnia, excessive worry, and obsessive-compulsive disorder (OCD).[12] It turns out that our feelings are largely controlled by the balance of bacteria in our gut and how they impact our brain via the vagus nerve, which connects the two. Suffice it to say this gives a whole new meaning to "gut feelings"; the ever-prescient Hippocrates noted centuries ago that there's an association between what you eat and how you feel.

Even our sleep can be impacted by these invisible bugs, which isn't all that surprising when you consider the fact that gut bacteria and sleep both play into our health in profound ways.[13] Here's the connection: Specialized biological molecules called cytokines are required to bring on sleep, particularly deep, restorative sleep. New research is showing that gut bacteria stimulate production of these chemicals in sync with cortisol levels. You've probably heard of cortisol, our body's main stress hormone. Levels of this hormone are tied to our circadian rhythm, changes in the body that follow a roughly twenty-four-hour cycle, responding primarily to light and darkness in the environment. Such changes determine whether we're feeling alert or tired. Cortisol should be lowest at night and begin to rise in the early morning hours. So these cytokines essentially have circadian cycles dictated by the gut bacteria. In the morning, when cortisol levels go up, these cytokines are inhibited, which defines the transition between sleep phases. Disruption of the gut bacteria can have major negative effects on sleep and circadian rhythms.

Let me give you one more wild example. Surgical approaches to weight loss, such as gastric bypass to physically change the digestive system, have become increasingly popular solutions to obesity. These procedures often involve making the stomach smaller and rerouting parts of the small intestine. We used to think that they triggered rapid weight loss largely by forcing the person to eat less, but another landmark study published in *Nature* in 2014 showed that the microbiome contributes to the success of gastric surgery.[14] A major portion of the weight loss is attributable to changes in the gut microbiota, changes that occur after surgery in response to not just the anatomical adjustments but the dietary shifts that typically happen as the person consumes foods that favor the growth of different bacteria. These patients often see a reversal in their diabetes as well soon after surgery, and I bet that part of that is also due to the changes in the composition of the gut bacteria.

A 2012 study published in *Science* found a link between a certain strain of bacteria (*E. coli*) disturbing the intestinal microbiome and causing colorectal cancer:

> Ecologists have long known that when some major change disturbs an environment in some way, ecosystem structure is likely

to change dramatically. Further, this shift in interconnected species' diversity, abundances, and relationships can in turn have a transforming effect on the health of the whole landscape—causing a rich woodland or grassland to become permanently degraded, for example—as the ecosystem becomes unstable and then breaks down the environment. For this reason, it should come as no surprise that a significant disturbance in the human body can profoundly alter the makeup of otherwise stable microbial communities coexisting within it and that changes in the internal ecology known as the human microbiome can result in unexpected and drastic consequences for human health.[15]

Once again, we see the power of context. Bacteria were earth's first inhabitants. In 2013, the oldest signs of life on earth—3.5 billion years old—were discovered in a remote region of northwest Australia, where evidence of a complex microbial ecosystem is locked in ancient rock formations. It was part of our evolution to forge a symbiotic relationship with bacteria.

The science of understanding the microbiome is still in its infancy, but I expect it will explode in the coming decade. We'll soon begin to understand how different microbiotic profiles, much like genetic profiles, are related to certain diseases or to optimal health. And we will begin to learn how we can leverage the microbiome to prevent and treat a variety of ailments, from neurodevelopmental challenges in early life to neurodegenerative problems and chronic illnesses in later life. You'll be able to figure out whether your gut is harboring tribes that code for wellness or, conversely, sickness. And you will be able to make targeted tweaks to your diet and daily habits to support the growth and maintenance of the right kind of microbes for you. You may think that you're doomed to have X, Y, and Z due to your genetics, but in the Lucky Years your fate will hinge more on how you play the cards you've been dealt through how you live than on solely which cards you hold.

All this goes to show that it's not all about human DNA, but about the microbiome, too. Our context comprises this dynamic duo. They may even complement each other in unexpected ways. For example, fully one-fifth of all genes in blood cells undergo seasonal changes in expression. This was just discovered during an elegant study performed by a couple of scientists at the University of Cambridge. They found that in the winter, your blood has a denser mix of immune responders.[16] And in the summer months, your blood contains more of the hormones that help the body to burn fat, build tissues, and retain water. These seasonal changes could offer insights into inflammatory diseases such as hypertension and autoimmune diseases such as type 1 diabetes. And such seasonal changes also occur in the microbiome, which in turn impacts health and risk for illness. Perhaps we will soon know, by virtue of the month or time of year, which genes are turning on and which microbes are dominating. This information can then tell us, in real time, what risks we face and which behaviors we should embrace to optimize our genetic and microbial machinery.

It's one thing to talk about sequencing genes and tumors, deleting our diseases, and learning about the human microbiome. But it's clearly another to bring the lessons of these technologies home to our everyday lives. So with that in mind, let me help you measure and interpret your own data. But before doing so, I want to give you a primer question to consider that will help you contextualize your life:

What are your personal health goals?

You've obviously picked up this book for a reason. So it helps to have a clear sense of your personal health goals as you proceed. And I hope they are loftier and more precise than just "I want to lose weight," or "I want to feel and look better." Aim higher with things like "I want to be able to play with my kids and grandkids when I'm older," or "I want to optimize my life today using the best medicine has to offer so I can reach my health goals now and in the future," or "I want to free myself from chronic anxiety and fear of the future so I can perform better at work and be more present and happy at home."

Now let's get personal.

CHAPTER 5

Take the Two-Week Challenge

How to Measure and Interpret Your Own Data

Observe, record, tabulate, communicate. Use your five senses.
Learn to see, learn to hear, learn to feel, learn to smell, and know
that by practice alone you can become expert.

—Sir William Osler

76 years	81 years	3.5 years	4.5 years	10 to 15 years
Life expectancy for men in the US	Life expectancy for women in the US	Curing cancer adds to life expectancy	Curing heart disease adds to life expectancy	Curing all major diseases adds to life expectancy

These data represent the hope for health prevention studies.

How long do you think you will live? How long do you *want* to live? How old are you biologically today, and how long will you live strong and happily, unencumbered by an illness or chronic condition?

The numbers in the chart above are real, and troubling to me. I can hardly stand the fact that many of my patients probably could have prevented their suffering from cancer or other life-altering diseases had they done a few things differently earlier in life. Kept their weight under control. Managed stress better. Quit smoking sooner. Made physical activity a regular habit. Been more attuned to what their bodies were telling them and acted accordingly. Stopped procrastinating on important tests and early-detection screenings.

Most of the data we have on file are observational. Scientists look at a large group of people—some of whom practiced one behavior and others another—and then they study the outcomes, attempting to make the groups equal with respect to other variables, with men and women of roughly the same age in each group, who share similar lifestyles in terms of their diet and exercise habits. These large, randomized controlled trials are the best resource we have to identify behaviors that can alter our risk for disease. The problem is that it is very hard to dictate behavior to a group of people and expect them to be compliant for years and then study an outcome that has a very long lag time, meaning time until the desired effect is seen. Few, if any, scientists want to stake their efforts and career on an experiment that won't yield a result for a decade or more. Which is why we need to discover shorter-term endpoints. For example, if we have a simple blood test for inflammation of the arteries, which leads to heart disease, we could have someone change a behavior and see how it affected that variable in the short term.

When HIV was spreading and patients had long been panicking by the late 1980s and early 1990s, scientists were developing drugs with the hope that they would change long-term outcomes of the disease. Traditional trials would have taken years to see such an effect, though, and no one had the luxury of time amid the epidemic. A clever group of lab scientists developed a blood test that counted first how many of the CD4 T cells were present in the patient. HIV targets these cells, and they plummet when the virus is active, leading to AIDS. Later a more accurate test was developed that counted how many copies of the virus are in the bloodstream. These are called surrogate markers, and in 1992 the FDA actually adopted new regulations (after much lobbying by the HIV patient advocates) designed to speed approval of important new treatments using these surrogate markers. The new regulation became known as the Accelerated Approval provisions. The FDA for the first time articulated an explicit requirement for drug approval based on the effect of a drug on a surrogate marker, and not just a clinical outcome. The key portion of the regulation reads as follows:

> The United States Food and Drug Administration (FDA) may grant marketing approval for a new drug product on the basis of adequate and well-controlled clinical trials establishing that the drug product has an effect on a surrogate endpoint that is reasonably likely, based on epidemiologic, therapeutic, patho-physiologic, or other evidence, to predict clinical benefit, or on the basis of an effect on a clinical endpoint other than survival or irreversible morbidity.[1]

This new legislation set the bar for developing drugs for a surrogate marker, and the number of HIV drugs in development exploded. The progress and excitement over these new drugs were palpable at the time. I remember being in the "Osler 8" medical ward at Hopkins, the place for patients who have infectious diseases (and most of the patients at this time had AIDS). The daily talk on rounds was about new data on these new drugs. Everyone, patients included, would discuss the new drugs and their progress in the clinic. I get excited when I think about what could happen if we developed validated surrogate markers for other diseases. There would be a dramatic increase in the development of drugs that could potentially delay or prevent diseases.

Although we've made huge strides in prolonging our life spans, we haven't yet necessarily done so well at staving off diseases that come with age—especially the chronic ones such as diabetes, heart disease, stroke, and cancer. So we're living longer, yes, but suffering through illnesses that can be debilitating and enormously diminishing to one's quality of life. In the United States alone, the number of people with chronic conditions is projected to increase steadily for the next thirty years. My hope is that we can curb this trend in the Lucky Years.

Today, these are the ten leading causes of death in the United States:

- heart disease
- cancer
- chronic lower-respiratory diseases (emphysema and chronic bronchitis)
- stroke
- unintentional injuries (accidents)
- Alzheimer's disease
- diabetes
- influenza and pneumonia
- kidney disease
- suicide

Infectious diseases such as tuberculosis, pneumonia, and diarrheal disease were the leading causes of death worldwide at the dawn of the twentieth century. By the beginning of the twenty-first century, in most of the developed world, death from communicable illnesses had been replaced by death from chronic illnesses that weren't necessarily blamed on a germ. Of all the causes of death in the United States, the leading top ten account for nearly 75 percent of all deaths, and the top three killers—heart disease, cancer, and lower-respiratory diseases—cause over 50 percent of all deaths.

Multimorbidity is the most common chronic condition today. This refers to the coexistence of multiple chronic diseases or conditions. Only 17 percent of people who have heart disease, for example, suffer from only that condition. The majority (almost 3 in 4) of individuals aged sixty-five years and older suffer from several chronic conditions, as do 1 in 4 adults younger than sixty-five years who receive health care. Adults with multiple chronic conditions are the chief users of health care services and account for the vast majority of health care spending.[2]

In all honesty, I don't know what true health is, particularly on an individual basis. For person A, health can be living totally free of illness

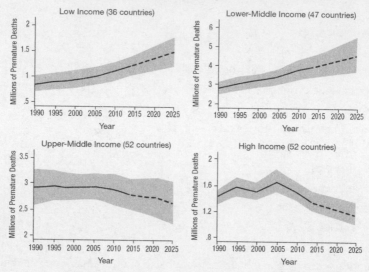

Premature (Under Age Sixty) Deaths from NCDs

There has been a rise in noncommunicable disease in low- and middle-income countries, due to advances in the treatment and prevention of communicable diseases. At the same time, there was a decrease in noncommunicable disease in the higher-income countries.

and disability. For person B, however, perhaps health means managing a condition well and enjoying life to the fullest despite some disability. While we can certainly try to measure health in a variety of ways—weight, cholesterol, blood sugar, blood cell count, hormone levels, markers of inflammation, how you look, and how well you sleep, for example—none of those figures or generalizations will tell the whole picture. And they won't reveal how many years and days you might have left on this planet.

Such a challenge is partly why I encourage you to view your total health as a complex network of processes that cannot be explained by looking at any one pathway or focal point. Health is in perpetual flux. You need to adapt to changes as you age, a message I've been driving home since the beginning. As I also noted earlier, in science-speak we say that humans are "emergent systems"—we are constantly changing,

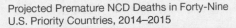

Projected Premature NCD Deaths in Forty-Nine
U.S. Priority Countries, 2014–2015

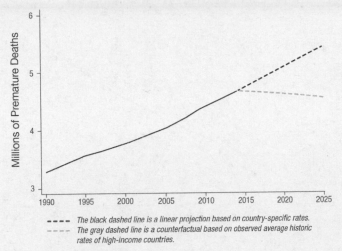

The black dashed line is a linear projection based on country-specific rates.
The gray dashed line is a counterfactual based on observed average historic
rates of high-income countries.

There are too many deaths from noncommunicable diseases in U.S. priority countries (the forty-nine countries in which the United States devoted five million dollars or more in aid for health in 2013). Noncommunicable disease accounted for 28 percent of the premature (under age sixty) deaths in these countries. That rate was 3.5 times greater than premature deaths from HIV/AIDS and 1.6 times as many premature deaths as malaria, tuberculosis (TB), and HIV/AIDS combined. The gray line represents what would happen if this trend followed the trends in high income countries.

developing, and evolving. The body is an incredible self-regulating machine. You don't need to do much to support its health and optimal wellness. In the last hour, for instance, about one billion cells were replaced in your body without your having to think about it. Our goal should be not only to maximize our life spans, but also to delay the onset of chronic diseases so we can make the last years or decades of life as fulfilling as possible.

Of all the lessons I like to give when I present to a large audience, the top three are: (1) record your body's features; (2) measure yourself; and (3) automate your life. What exactly do I mean by these recommendations? To start with, I'll talk about one of the biggest hurdles we all face in making our lives better: honesty.

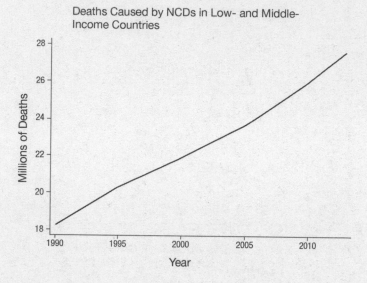

Deaths Caused by NCDs in Low- and Middle-Income Countries

The death rate from noncommunicable disease in low- and middle-income countries is growing at a disconcerting pace, especially among the poorest populations. This is an epidemic.

Time to Get Real

About 67 percent of Americans are overweight or obese, a statistic that you've no doubt heard over and over again. But only 36 percent of these individuals admit to being overweight. And the others don't admit it because *they don't know it.* In other words, they may not be in denial; they might be so out of touch with their own reality that they cannot recognize and accept the fact that they are overweight.

Indeed, this finding is counterintuitive: we assume that everyone is aware of obesity, including those who are overweight. The fact that someone could be overweight or obese and not know it seems unbelievable, as if you grew an extra limb and didn't notice. But this phenomenon is not news to health professionals. I routinely treat patients who don't recognize how overweight they are or who minimize their weight as just "a few extra pounds."

A 2010 study published in the journal *Obstetrics & Gynecology* turned conventional wisdom on its head when it reported that nearly 40 percent of overweight women and a little more than 10 percent of obese women believed themselves to be of normal weight or underweight.[3] The general media has us thinking that most women perceive themselves as fat, but the same study showed that only 16 percent of normal-weight women in the study saw themselves as overweight. One of the study's authors makes a good point: when the world around you is obese, you begin to identify overweight as normal, and this thinking is not based on the scale but on how you simply perceive yourself in your context.[4]

And it's not just excess fat that people are oblivious to: nearly two-thirds of parents underestimate their children's weight. According to a study published in 2014 in the journal *Pediatrics*, half of parents don't even see that their children are overweight or obese.[5] What's more, about 30 percent of kids and teens ages eight to fifteen misperceive their own weight status. Among children and teens who were deemed overweight by medical standards (between the 85th and 95th percentiles on the CDC's growth chart), 76 percent thought they were "about right"; approximately 23 percent said they were overweight. Among obese kids and teens (those in the 95th percentile and higher on the chart), about 42 percent thought they were okay weight-wise, while 57 percent believed they were in the "overweight" category. Younger kids, boys, and children from poorer families were more likely to misperceive their weight.[6]

Our reluctance to acknowledge our weight problems affects our health tremendously. For example, breast cancer is the most common cancer among women, and postmenopausal obese women are nearly 60 percent more likely to develop this cancer compared to their healthy-weight counterparts. Ignorance may be bliss in some circumstances, but in many areas of health, ignorance can be deadly.

The idea that we tend to disregard or underestimate our own risk factors for health conditions extends far beyond matters of weight. How many of us, for instance, miscalculate how much processed sugar we consume, how much exercise we get, and how much stress we are under? We're terrible at self-evaluating these important metrics and keeping them in check. A recent landmark study shows a huge gap between how much sugar people think they consume and the reality. And the reality is more dramatically skewed the more overweight a person gets. Put another way, obese individuals are more likely than people of normal weight to underestimate their sugar consumption significantly.

In this particular study, a team of scientists from the universities of Reading and Cambridge, in the United Kingdom, and Arizona State University compared sugar intake in 1,700 people.[7] They used two methods: self-reported sugar consumption and sugar levels in urine samples, the latter of which was the more accurate and objective measure. After three years, those taking part in the study had their body mass index (BMI) measured. The researchers found that the people who ate the most sugar, as determined using the urine test, were 54 percent more likely to be overweight than those who ate less sugar. And obese participants tended to misrepresent how much sugar they were consuming. The people who claimed to be eating the most sugar were actually 44 percent less likely to be obese than those who said they were consuming the lowest amounts.

Granted, this study had its limitations, and many other variables were likely involved to arrive at these results. We cannot, for example, conclude that sugar causes obesity from this one investigation. But we can entertain the fact that we each have an underlying psychology at play when it comes to accepting our behaviors. Such a psychology can work for or against us. Which brings me to the two-week challenge. It's time to get real. It's time to take an honest look at where—and who—you are in matters of health.

The Two-Week Challenge

Two weeks. I'm going to ask you to work through this chapter over the course of fourteen days. You may even gain benefits that you feel physically toward the end of these two weeks. The whole point here is to help you identify your own personal context and then optimize that context going forward with the information in the coming chapters. And this exercise won't require a doctor's appointment, although I will give you some tips to maximize the benefit of your next doctor's visit. Here's what you will need:

- Pen and paper (or computer file; basically, a way to keep track of what you're doing over these next fourteen days)
- A way to measure your blood pressure (you can buy these devices at local pharmacies or online)

To remind you of the analogy I used before: If I asked you to tell me how long it takes to drive from New York to Los Angeles, some of the questions you will ask are which roads are taken, which type of car is driven, even who is driving. You can take the car apart and examine all of the pieces individually but still can't tell how long it will take to get to the destination. There are just too many variables—and the same is true of the complex human body. No one can tell you how long it'll go on cruise control before hitting a roadblock or meeting its endpoint. But there are big factors that play mightily into health that should be considered. This is akin to telling you that the drive in a modern car from A to B will cover 2,500 miles on major highways under excellent driving and weather conditions. With that kind of contextual information, you have more data to predict the experience. I want you to have that kind of data in terms of your health, so you can have the best experience down your own road in life. Below are the top ten factors—your car parts—that can help you achieve just that.

Factor 1: Chronological Age
The decade you are in today automatically provides a lot of context. A person in her thirties, for example, will have a different set of health issues and concerns than someone in her sixties. Time goes by fast for most of us, and we can easily lose sight of what we should be considering health-wise, just based on our age alone. We may feel thirty

when we're sixty, but that doesn't mean our bones and metabolism are behaving as such.

Obviously, the risk of developing age-related chronic disease increases as you get older. One of the invisible lines seems to be around the age of forty, after which the body begins to go through more dramatic shifts as it moves out of the fertile years, and it becomes more important to stay on top of certain screenings. This is also the time when taking more aggressive preventive measures such as a baby aspirin a day and/or a statin should be considered. The importance of establishing healthy habits in your twenties and thirties cannot be overstated. Chronic disease doesn't happen spontaneously when you're older. It's the accumulation of insults to the body over time, coupled with underlying genes, that often result in illness later in life. The problem is that it's very difficult to think about the health challenges of aging when you're young or enjoying great health. But planning for optimal health is just as important as planning for future financial needs.

Whatever decade of life you're in, I encourage you to check your blood pressure twice daily over the next two weeks. See if you can find a pattern to it. Does it go up after lunch and down after exercise? Check it at different times throughout the fourteen days, and note what's going on during those times ("just woke up" or "just had an argument with my teenage son"). This experiment will help you identify your blood pressure range, so months or even years from now you can tell if that range has shifted—for better or worse.

Factor 2: Heritage and Family History

Do you know what killed your great-grandparents on both sides of the family? Or what kind of cancer your uncle Elroy had when he was forty? Family history is one of the most underused but extremely powerful tools to understanding your health. And it may be the best tool to predict genetic cancer risks. Good family health trees are rare; less than a third of us have one, and my bet is your doctor hasn't pushed you to complete your family tree (despite those questions you tried to fill out during your first visit).

The US Surgeon General operates a free website—https://family history.hhs.gov—that will help you to create a family health history, learn about your risk for conditions that can run in families, and share it electronically with relatives and your doctor. Be sure to include as much information from both sides of the family as possible, and record any environmental or lifestyle factors that could have contributed to a family member's untimely death. Who smoked? Who was overweight? Who was hospitalized or treated for mental illness? The answers to these questions can be enlightening on many levels and can lead to better personal care. Once you exhaust the limits of this kind of rough detective work, you may want to consider taking it to the next level and undergo genetic screening. But remember that DNA tests aren't as much of an oracle into your future risks and health as you might think, and they are not for everyone.

Factor 3: Daily Patterns and Habits

A popular children's book, *Eat, Sleep, Poop*, has more to say about life and health than you might think. Babies are born with an inherent programming to know what they require to survive. They have distinct patterns to their needs, which are dictated primarily by the urge to eat, sleep, and poop and pee. We as adults often don't listen to and follow our bodies' physiological cues and needs for the very same fundamental activities. We can let distractions and responsibilities rule our lives, as well as wield the power of the mind over matter.

One of the most important things to know about your body is that it loves rhythms, patterns, and predictability. There is a reason we tend to get tired at the same time each day, to wake up within the same fifteen minutes each morning, to crave coffee at the same time, and to feel hunger for dinner at about the same time every day. Maintaining such routines reduces stress on the body and keeps its preferred, balanced state of being—a state in medicine we call homeostasis. Another way of understanding homeostasis is to consider the human body's average temperature of 98.6 degrees F. When it shoots up, it's a sign that something is wrong or out of balance inside, perhaps set off by an infection. The body then goes to work on remedying the problem to bring down the temperature back to normal. It does this all day long based on what you encounter and how you treat your body to either support its natural balance or challenge it.

To get a sense of how powerful timing can be for the body, look no further than a study done in 2015 and published in the prestigious journal *Science*.[8] Researchers at San Diego State University and the Salk Institute for Biological Studies discovered that by limiting the period during which fruit flies could eat, they could prevent heart problems related to diet and aging. They also found that genes responsible for circadian rhythm—the body's internal clock that's aligned with the twenty-four-hour solar day—are integral to this process.

As with mice, fruit flies have long been used as model organisms to study the genetic basis of human disease, including cardiovascular disease. The average life span of a fruit fly is about thirty days, thereby making experiments on aging and disease even easier. Fruit flies share with us a number of genes that control development of a complex, symmetrical body plan. Thomas Hunt Morgan and his students at Columbia University identified the first fruit fly mutations in the early 1900s. Ever since, scientists have amassed an extensive library of genetic mutants for study. It's easy to play with fruit fly genes, disrupting them or introducing foreign ones. This is what makes the fruit fly such a versatile and excellent model organism for studying animal development, including behavior, learning, and memory.

From previous research, we already knew that late-night eaters are more prone to developing heart disease than those who stop eating earlier. But this study adds a lot more to the notion that timing can mean everything. More specifically, here's what these clever researchers did. In their experiments, one group of young fruit flies was fed freely a standard diet of cornmeal (the flies could eat to their hearts' content all day long). Another group had only a twelve-hour daily window during which they could access the food.

Over the next several weeks, the scientists recorded the food consumption among the flies. They also checked a slew of health param-

eters related to their sleep, body weight, and heart physiology. At the
three-week mark, the results were in: flies limited to eating within the
twelve-hour time frame slept better, didn't pack on as much weight,
and had far healthier hearts than their "eat anytime" peers. This was
true even though both groups consumed similar amounts of food. After
five weeks, the researchers documented the same results. In fact, the
difference between the hearts of the twelve-hour eaters versus those
eating all twenty-four were so striking that the researchers thought for a
moment that they had mistaken some young three-week-old flies for the
older group. They repeated the experiments several times to convince
themselves that, indeed, the improvement was related to the time-
limited feeding. Moreover, another set of experiments showed that the
young flies weren't the only ones benefiting from a time-restricted diet.
The older flies' hearts became healthier when they were forced to eat
only during a twelve-hour period daily. So even if you limit the feeding
starting very late in the life cycle, there are still some benefits, and they
can persist. In these experiments, even the flies that went back to eating
whenever they wanted still enjoyed some degree of heart protection.

What's the underlying mechanism here? How can *when* you eat have
such a biological impact despite the amount or quality of the calories?
To answer this, the scientists dug into the genetics. At various points
in the experiment they sequenced the flies' RNA to see which of their
genes had been turned on or off as a result of time-restricted feeding.
For the record, ribonucleic acid, or RNA, is one of the three major
biological macromolecules that are essential for all known forms of
life (along with DNA and proteins). The flow of genetic information
in a cell is from DNA through RNA to proteins: "DNA makes RNA
makes protein," hence studying the RNA of a species can show which
genes are turned on or off. In this particular study, the researchers
identified three genetic pathways that seem to be involved in these
gene expression changes: the TCP-1 ring complex chaperonin, which
helps proteins fold; mitochondrial electron transport chain complexes
(mETC), which relate to the energy cycle of a cell; and a collection of
genes in charge of the body's circadian rhythm.

Then the scientists repeated their experiments with flies that carried mutations in their DNA that adversely affected their TCP-1 and circadian rhythm genes. In these flies, time-limited feeding conferred no health benefits, further suggesting that these genetic pathways play important parts. In the flies with the modified mETC genes, however, twelve-hour feeding showed enhanced protection against cardiac aging.

Although science has yet to understand fully how these three pathways work together to increase or decrease risk of cardiovascular conditions, one thing is clear: daily eating patterns can have a profound impact on our bodies, including our brains, where the entire circadian rhythm is literally clocked. These results actually complement earlier research showing benefits of time-restricted feeding for obesity, metabolic diseases, and type 2 diabetes in rodents.

So the message is clear: time does matter. The three chief areas where you can make great strides in honoring your body's homeostasis are your eating times, sleep-wake cycles, and periods of physical activity. If you take medications, scheduling that to occur at the same time daily is also important. And that's what you're going to do over the next fourteen days: keep track of these daily routines. I don't expect every single day to be identical to the next, but see if you can create a consistent pattern that's more or less the same on a daily basis. Below is a sample entry for two different days, with notes added at the end of each day:

Wake up / go to bed: 6:30 a.m. / 10:30 p.m.
Exercise: 7:00 a.m.
Eating: 8:00 a.m.; 11:00 a.m. (snack); 1:00; 4:00 (snack); 7 p.m.
Note: 11:00 snack unusual (office birthday party)

Wake up / go to bed: 6:30 a.m. / 11:00 p.m.
Exercise: none
Eating: 7:30 a.m.; 12:00; 3:00 (snack); 7 p.m.
Note: didn't feel as good in the afternoon; took Tylenol for
    headache.

You can track a lot more than these basics, but this will give you a good start. The goal is to record the most prominent activities in your daily life that repeat on a twenty-four- to forty-eight-hour cycle, which for most are at least these three items. Note any nuances or deviations.

Factor 4: Weight and Dietary Preferences

Do you have a plant-based diet? Or would you call yourself a bona fide carnivore? Is your weight in an ideal place today, or could you lose a few pounds, perhaps twenty? How many times have you tried to lose weight permanently via a popular diet protocol? Do you even know what you weigh and if it's within a healthy range for your height?

It should come as no surprise that carrying excess weight can sabotage the body's optimal functionality, especially in the absence of cardiorespiratory fitness. Being overweight increases your risk for most illnesses and chronic conditions, from the obvious ones such as heart disease and diabetes, to dementia and cancer.

If you don't know how much you weigh, get yourself on a scale to find out your poundage and then plug that number into an online body mass index calculator, which is a general measure of body fat based on height and weight. The National Heart, Lung, and Blood Institute has an easy-to-use calculator at https://www.nhlbi.nih.gov/health /educational/lose_wt/BMI/bmicalc.htm. An ideal BMI for most people is between 18.5 and 24.9, although there is some wiggle room if you're physically fit and have a naturally larger body frame and carry extra muscle mass, which will push your BMI higher due to the weight of that muscle. By some standards, a BMI of 26 or 27 isn't too terrible if you don't have any metabolic conditions such as signs of diabetes and you're in excellent physical shape.

There is no such thing as the "best diet." The best one is the one that works for your physiology. And even though we have studies to show that, for example, a Mediterranean diet can reduce the risk of various diseases and decrease mortality, by no means is it the only diet. Also keep in mind that there's no such thing as *the* Mediterranean diet. It just has some universal features: plenty of whole fruits, vegetables, whole grains, legumes, nuts, and seeds; fat from healthy sources like olive oil; a little bit of dairy, fish, poultry, and eggs; a smaller bit of red meat; and maybe a glass of wine with dinner. How can you argue with that?

We all can agree that any traditional diet will beat our processed-food culture. Just about every food fad of late, including the Paleo or primal diet, has been flawed (our Paleolithic ancestors didn't just gnaw on meat all day; new evidence from the dental plaque of early Paleolithic people, dating back 400,000 years ago, shows they enjoyed a balanced diet including plants, nuts, and seeds).[9] Traditional eating habits have worked for centuries among different cultures with vastly different diets around the world. But they do have a lot in common, such as moderate portions, communal eating, and letting hunger build in between meals (no grazing or snacking). Only in recent times have people begun to demonize certain ingredients or whole categories of food. The top five that I continually hear about are sugar, gluten (and wheat in general), dairy, alcohol, and red meat. Let's dissect the dispute about red meat, which I should remind you has been a staple in many cultures for centuries.

A couple of years ago, researchers at the Harvard School of Public Health came out with a study linking red meat and death. It got the media talking, to say the least. You probably read the alarming headlines: "Red Meat Death Study" and "Will Red Meat Kill You?" According to the study, the results of which were published in no less an authority than the *Archives of Internal Medicine* (now called *JAMA Internal Medicine*), for every extra serving above and beyond an acceptable single serving of unprocessed red meat consumed daily (think steak, hamburger, pork, etc.) the risk of dying prematurely went up by 13 percent.[10] Processed red meat, including hot dogs, bacon, and sausage, increased the risk by 20 percent.

This was no small study, either. It included data from more than 37,000 men involved in the Health Professionals Follow-up Study, and 83,600 women from the Nurses' Health Study. These volunteers were followed for an average of twenty-four years, during which 23,926 of them died. Every four years, these participants submitted information about their diets. The people who ate the most red meat had higher death rates compared to those who ate the least. To date, this has been the largest, longest study on the alleged link between red meat and life span. While the findings have merit, these numbers do need to be put into perspective—and brought into the right context.

The same year of the Harvard study (2012), a Japanese investigation that looked at more than 51,000 men and women over the course of sixteen years failed to find a connection between meat consumption and premature death.[11] In 2010, another study by different researchers from the Harvard School of Public Health also found no connection between unprocessed red meat and the development of heart disease and diabetes. But they did find a strong relationship with *processed* red meat.[12]

Now let's review some numbers. If red meat increases your risk of dying by 13 percent or 20 percent, that might motivate you to ignore your cravings for a juicy steak and learn to love tofu, or eat just chicken and fish. But don't forget that we're talking about relative risks. When scientists make these comparisons, they look at death rates in people eating the least meat with those eating the most. So it behooves us to consider the absolute risks, which paint a different and much more comforting picture.[13]

According to the authors of the *Archives* paper, the increased risk from red meat is likely multifactorial. It could be due to the saturated fat, cholesterol, and iron that meat contains. It could be partially due to the effects from cooking red meat at high temperatures, which can produce potentially cancer-causing compounds. There also could be a potential driver in red meat's sodium content, particularly in processed foods. Moreover, we can't ignore the fact that major red-meat eaters often have other risk factors for serious, life-shortening diseases. While stereotypical, there is data to show that people who eat too much red meat also have a propensity to shun exercise, drink excessively, and use tobacco. Put simply, a lot of variables are in the mix; things are not always what they seem to be on the surface. An important conclusion by the researchers is their estimate that 9.3 percent of deaths in men and 7.6 percent in women could have been prevented at the end of the study period if all the participants had consumed less than 0.5 servings per day of red meat. That is three and a half servings per week. Moderation is the key here. Meat isn't necessarily bad, but too much meat and processed meat are bad.

While this moderation principle should be obvious to any well-read individual, far too often, we're out of touch with what—and how much—we're eating. Perhaps you think you are eating well when in actuality you're exceeding the recommended limits for sugar, fat, and salt three days a week. Over the next fourteen days, aim to record your eating habits. Try to be as precise as possible, recording amounts, quality, and types of, say, fat and protein. Distinguish between a meal from McDonald's and a homemade burger with grass-fed beef, or a green salad with olive oil versus a Cobb salad with commercially made ranch dressing. Include beverages, from water, juice, and milk, to wine, liquor, and beer. Which foods make you feel good within the hours afterward and the next day? Which choices render you sluggish, achy, or moody?

Remember, there's a connection between the food you eat and how you feel. By keeping a food diary, you can quickly see how your choices are impacting you and where you can make adjustments. The goal is to see where your diet may be lacking or overly abundant. Don't worry about trying to count calories or grams of nutrients. I trust you'll be able to see easily where your diet could be improved using common sense. This exercise also might help you pinpoint foods that make you feel especially good or bad. Make any additional notes as you see fit.

Factor 5: Medications and Management of Conditions

How many pills do you take a day, prescription or otherwise? Do you know exactly what each drug is for and why you take it? Do you manage a chronic condition through these drugs alone? Do you know if there are additional ways to manage your condition aside from drugs? If, for example, you're a diabetic, do you still watch your diet and commit to an exercise routine? If, for another example, you're a marathoner who trains hard on the weekend, do you find yourself taking upwards of ten over-the-counter pain relievers to combat the muscle aches? What about vitamins and supplements? Do you know why you take them if you do, and if you really need them? Or could they be harming you in ways you don't realize?

One of my favorite quotes by Sir William Osler is "The person who takes medicine must recover twice, once from the disease and once from the medicine." Don't get me wrong: drugs—prescription and nonprescription—do have their place in medicine and health. But it's true that far too many people rely on them for the wrong reasons. In 2013, a study from Mayo Clinic researchers revealed the depth of our drug dependency: 7 out of 10 Americans take at least one prescription drug; more than half of Americans take two prescription medications, and 20 percent of Americans are on at least five prescription medications.[14] Although we'd like to think these drugs are prescribed for the most common chronic conditions—heart disease and diabetes—it turns out that antibiotics are the most prescribed drugs; they are taken by 17 percent of Americans, followed by antidepressants and opioids, each taken by 13 percent of Americans. Clearly, this goes to show how mental health is a huge issue that we should focus on. Prescriptions for antidepressants are more common among women than among men, especially among women ages fifty to sixty-four, nearly 25 percent of which take these drugs.

So here's your challenge: take inventory of your medications and the conditions for which they are prescribed. Also include the over-the-counter drugs, vitamins, and supplements you take and why you take them. You may find that you can't fully answer the *why* part. And you may feel inspired to taper off certain medications and supplements or find alternative ways to manage your condition that are better for you and your body. Let me give you one quick example: A friend of mine realized she was taking up to thirty ibuprofen tablets weekly to manage a foot problem she had that plagued her during the day, especially with exercise. When she started to experience gastrointestinal issues and a slight decrease in her kidney function linked to the ibuprofen, she was forced to stop and consider why her foot started hurting as soon as she rolled out of bed most mornings. After some visits to an orthopedic surgeon who specialized in feet, she learned that she had a degenerative condition in one of her foot joints that had been caused by trauma many years back. She had a surgical procedure on the joint, which after a recovery period led her to being ibuprofen-free. She changed her context. I can give story after story here, but the realization of context is the unifying theme.

Don't underestimate those over-the-counter medications, many of which were once prescriptions. I'm glad to see the FDA strengthening the warning labels on popular OTC pain relievers. These commonly used drugs are not risk-free; they increase the risk of heart-related problems with regular use and can do so within a matter of weeks.

Factor 6: Unexplained Symptoms

Over the two-week challenge, make sure to record any unexplained symptoms you have that are out of the ordinary. They can be any number of things: feelings of nausea or stomach upset, a night sweat, an achy back or sore joint, an intense thirst, or the urge to nap on a Tuesday afternoon when you never nap. These symptoms are probably absolutely nothing to worry about, but they can nonetheless clue you in to signs that make up part of your context.

Factor 7: Sleep Needs

How many hours of sleep a night do you typically get? Is this enough? Do you ever suffer from insomnia or rely on sleep aids?

Although we used to think for a long time that a typical adult needs between seven and nine hours of sleep a night, newer research is showing that the magic number for most might be closer to seven, which is associated with the lowest mortality and morbidity. Other recent research has shown that a bad night's sleep, even losing a mere twenty minutes, can impair performance and memory the next day. We all know someone who claims to be fine on a few hours of sleep a night, but the research speaks otherwise, indicating that people who skimp on sleep many nights in a row don't perform as well on complex mental tasks as those who bank closer to seven hours a night. The research also says that getting less or much more than seven hours of sleep a night is associated with a higher mortality rate.[15] Sleep too much and you may be more prone to diabetes, obesity, and cardiovascular disease.

As we'll see in more detail in chapter 8, every system in the body is affected by the quality and amount of sleep you get per night. In fact, sleep directs so much of your body's physiological rhythms that you can't reboot yourself artificially with any substance or technology. You need a regular, reliable pattern of wakefulness and rejuvenating sleep to refresh your cells and tissues, to support your hardworking immune system, and to regulate your hormones. Which is why the proven benefits are plentiful: sleep can dictate how much you eat, how fat you get, whether you can fight off infections, how creative and insightful you can be, how well you can cope with stress, how fast you can process information, and how well you can store memories. The side effects of poor sleep habits are equally plentiful: hypertension, confusion, memory loss, chronic colds, the inability to learn new things, obesity, cardiovascular disease, and depression. So much of the body's natural rhythm that governs your health revolves around your sleep habits. When people complain of feeling tired and blue, I often start by asking them about their sleep schedule. It's the easiest way to regulate your body and feel a positive difference in a short time.

Question is, do you know how well you sleep? You should be able to figure out your optimal amount of sleep in a matter of days. Don't use an alarm clock. Go to sleep when you get tired. Stay off electronic devices as much as possible beforehand (and definitely keep them out of the room). If you do enjoy watching TV or videos on a device with a screen, as for some this can be relaxing prior to bedtime, get a pair of glasses that has a lens to block the brain-activating wavelengths of light. These blue-light blocking glasses are the cost of a large pizza. I put mine on when I have a chance to watch late-night comedy or the news before going to sleep. Track your sleep with a diary or a device that records your actual sleep time (lots of apps will help you track your sleep and circadian rhythm). If you feel refreshed and awake during the day, you've probably found your optimal sleep time.

Over these two weeks, in addition to finding your sleep number, document your sleep experience. Is it sound? Do you dream? If you do rely on sleep aids, be they over-the-counter drugs or prescription, can you make it a goal to wean yourself off of them? (Note that discontinuing some sleep aids may require the help of a doctor.)

Factor 8: Movement Matters

You already know that exercise does a body good. A daily brisk twenty-minute walk, for example, can reduce your risk of dying prematurely by a whopping 30 percent. Some studies say that a twenty-five-minute stroll can add seven years to life. How fast older people walk, in fact, is one of the most useful markers for determining future health. And it's just recently been shown that being sedentary may be twice as deadly as being obese. But I'll get to those details shortly. For now, it's time to get up close and personal with your exercise habits. How much do you move each day? How many consecutive hours do you sit? How many minutes do you get your heart rate up 50 percent above your resting baseline? Are you among the 82 percent of the 53 million Americans who belong to a gym but don't consistently use their membership?

Answer these questions over the next two weeks as you record your physical activity habits. If you work in a labor-intensive job, such as construction, or you are someone who is always on her feet running around taking care of things, you get extra points. You can track your activities using apps on your smartphone or a wearable fitness tracker (accelerometer), but this is optional. You can do just as well being tuned in to your activities and writing them down. Again, no need to try and calculate calories burned. Just write down how many minutes you were engaged in a physical activity and its intensity. Be as honest as possible. As with underestimating how much we eat, we also tend to underestimate our sedentary times while inflating our level of physical activity, and men are more likely than women to exaggerate.

Factor 9: Mood and Motivation

One of the most powerful questions a doctor can ask a patient is simply, "How do you feel?" Which can be a surprisingly difficult question to address personally. I wonder, if people were more attuned to their changing moods, behavioral triggers, and other aspects of their daily lives, would so many people be taking powerful mind-altering medications to regulate their moods?

Not only does tracking your mood help you better understand why symptoms occur when they do, but the information can also reveal whether drugs or therapy that you may be using are actually working. Mood monitoring can also help you find useful correlations, such as being predictably moody while talking to certain people or during the first half of the workweek when your blood pressure tends to run high, too.

Plenty of online mood trackers and apps are available today, but again, you can do this the old-fashioned way just by using your intuition about how you feel and making note of that. Track your mood throughout the day or during the same times you're testing your blood pressure.

Factor 10: Energy Levels

How is your energy level today on a scale of 1 to 5 (5 being the highest)? Do you feel full of life and ready to tackle any challenge (5)? Could you barely get out of bed (1)? Or are you somewhere in between?

A confluence of factors determine your energy level: how well you slept the night before, what you've been eating, how stressed you are, whether you're exercising too much or too little, and health conditions. While tracking energy levels is a little more amorphous than, say, logging your sleep time, see if you can find a pattern to your energy levels over these next two weeks. Maybe you'll discover that your body reaches a peak in energy at ten in the morning and then slowly wanes throughout the day. Or perhaps you'll question why your energy takes a dip at precisely four in the afternoon and then ticks up a notch again at five. All of these details fill in the blanks for your context and help you to make sense of your behaviors, and whether or not you want to change them.

Putting It All Together

Although this two-week challenge is not meant to be a scientific experiment, it can nonetheless uncover lots of things about you that you might not have known before or that you've simply ignored. All of this data will help you establish a new baseline for your health today, one that you can compare with future "checkpoints" during which you tune in to yourself and take stock of where you are in your overall health equation. You have listened to your body talk, and when you put each of the pieces together, there may be trends. Do you sleep better when you move more? Do you feel better when you have certain meals? And so on.

It always helps to have some lab work included in your data to create a fuller picture. And while you may not have any intention of going to the doctor today, below is an abbreviated list of the tests to ask for when you do:

- **Fasting lipid profile:** This test, which should be taken after twelve hours of fasting, gives you cholesterol (total cholesterol, HDL, and LDL values) and triglyceride numbers. A desirable total cholesterol is between 120 and 200 mg/dL, but this can be offset by a healthy ratio of good to bad cholesterol (more good HDL cholesterol and less bad LDL cholesterol). An ideal HDL level is greater than 60 mg/dL. An optimal LDL level is less than 100 mg/dL. Anything between 100 and 129 mg/dL is borderline, 130 to 159 mg/dL is considered mildly high, 160 to 189 is deemed moderately high, and an LDL level of 190 and above is severely high. A target triglyceride level is less than 150 mg/dL, with values between 150 and 199 being borderline, 200 to 499 being elevated, and values 500 and higher being severely elevated, placing one at high risk of the potentially deadly disease, pancreatitis, as well as heart disease. The recommended numbers for each of these lipid values are more stringent if you have previously documented heart disease.

- **High-sensitivity C-reactive protein (CRP):** This is a general marker of inflammation in the body, which can point to a number of potential problems and risk for disease. Higher levels are correlated with higher risk for a variety of illnesses and metabolic conditions, including diabetes, heart disease, and obesity. This number should be between 0.00 and 2.0 mg/L (ideally, less than 1.0).

- **Comprehensive metabolic panel (CMP):** You'll want this test to assess your liver, kidneys, electrolyte, and acid/base balance, and blood sugar and blood proteins.

- **Hemoglobin A1C:** Hemoglobin A1C (also called glycosylated hemoglobin) is the protein in red blood cells that carries oxygen. It also sticks to blood sugar, which is how measuring hemoglobin A1C can determine your blood sugar levels, and whether you're at risk for diabetes or already diabetic. This test is not a real-time measure of your blood sugar level; it reflects an "average" of your blood sugar levels over the previous ninety days (red blood cells live about that long). This is why studies of blood sugar control's possible role in various disease processes—from diabetes and heart disease to dementia—frequently use hemoglobin A1C. An ideal hemoglobin A1C is between 4.2 percent and 5.6 percent. Values of 5.7 percent to 6.4 percent indicate an increased risk for type 2 diabetes; values greater than or equal to 6.5 percent indicate type 2 diabetes. Your hemoglobin A1C number is not fixed; you can lower it through better nutrition and more physical exercise.

There's an inherent fear when you go look at your stock portfolio daily. But you're probably not so nervous when you look at it monthly. You can't look at it every day or you'd be trading too often. You need to treat your health like you treat your portfolio. You casually collect data over time and then go to a doctor and discuss it. Remember, you're looking at trends over time. I've asked you to scrutinize yourself pretty intensely for only two weeks. But you could just as easily extend that data collection period to a month or two or even three and be a little more casual about it. At the least, start to overlay blood pressure, weight, dietary patterns, sleeping habits, and so on, and see what emerges. If you give yourself more time to collect data, then you can even go so far as to play war games on yourself like I'm trying to do in the lab with a virtual tumor—a model of a cancer that can be manipulated in its environment to see what changes we can force on it to modify its behavior or growth. What if I mutated this gene? What if I exposed it to substance X?

Likewise, you might find yourself testing new methods in your own life. Maybe you'll spend four days avoiding the diet soda you love so much and see if that has any impact on your sleep and how you feel. Or maybe you'll realize that you feel your best on the days you get up at 6:15 sharp and don't lounge in bed until 7:00. These are the small details I hope you uncover about yourself. Have fun with this experiment. Next, we will learn more about how to add depth to your context and find what's right for you as you enter the Lucky Years.

CHAPTER 6

The Danger of Misinformation

How to Know Whom and What to Trust

The greater the ignorance, the greater the dogmatism.

—Sir William Osler

Pop quiz: Which of the following debates is, well, debatable?

   a. Vaccines can cause neurological disorders, including autism.
   b. Lifestyle habits can reverse cancer.
   c. Vitamins and supplements can boost your health.

Before I get to the answer (which would probably surprise you if I told you right now), let's take a tour of the current landscape in the dispensation of medical information. Every day I seem to encounter black-and-white, grandiose headlines in the media that I know must cause confusion and misinformation in the public. And some of the most egregious ones advertise a remedy or cure to our most difficult challenges, from depression and obesity to dementia and cancer. Or they peddle junk science, making declaratory statements and recommendations that are not backed by rigorous studies. Some of my favorites:

- Green coffee: miracle weight-loss cure in a bottle.
- Use this trick to look fifteen years younger.
- Dad discovers unique way to regrow hair.
- Diet cures cancer.
- Study: Placebo or not, acupuncture helps with pain.
- Vitamin E improves brainpower.
- Low vitamin D levels cause type 2 diabetes.
- Yoga and meditation can reverse heart disease.
- Chemicals in foods make you fat and sick and age you faster.
- Pasteurized milk is toxic.
- GMOs are toxic.
- Sugar is toxic.
- *You* are toxic!

Aspirational ideas are attractive. It's human nature to believe that there's a "secret" to being thinner, younger, sexier, smarter, and richer. While these beliefs can sometimes do us good, they can also lead us far astray from what's real and what's actually helpful. And a quick search online to decipher between truth and fiction might not help you out either. In 2014, a study published in the *Journal of the American Osteopathic Association* found significant errors in 9 out of 10 Wikipedia articles related to the ten most costly diseases and conditions in the United States, including coronary artery disease, major depression, diabetes, and back pain.[1] The study stated that Wikipedia has become a go-to source for health care information for both patients and practitioners, which isn't too surprising when you think about it. As I said, we all like swift resolutions, and Wikipedia is always a click away, usually at the top of the list of results to any search. But all sources, even peer-reviewed journals, can contain errors. You just cannot rely on any single source, no matter where it comes from.

Let's say, for a quick example, that you hear about saw palmetto being good for an enlarged prostate. It's advertised on television, in articles, and at your local pharmacy or market where supplements line a long aisle of organic wares. You think it's harmless but potentially beneficial. No one mentions side effects. And no one alerts you to the fact that saw palmetto changes the way the body metabolizes some drugs. It also slows blood clotting and acts like a hormone in the body. Once you begin to understand these nuances, a whole new picture emerges that's totally different from the one drawn in your head from advertising.

I always try to make conclusions based on good research, which typically means large-scale, double-blind, placebo-controlled studies that weed out certain variables and have conclusions that clearly reflect the results, are meaningful for people, and can be replicated by others in equally rigorous studies. Unfortunately, such studies are few and far between these days. And erroneous studies and conclusions can remain alive in the public imagination for many years despite new evidence to refute them. Look no further than the current debate about vaccines and autism, which was sparked by an unscrupulous doctor who published a bad study in a prestigious journal more than fifteen years ago.

You likely know some of the story. In 1998, a British doctor, Andrew Wakefield, announced that he had found a relationship between the MMR vaccine (for measles, mumps, rubella) and the development of autism. The MMR shot is usually administered to children at twelve months of age followed by a booster between ages four and six. According to Wakefield, who studied a scant twelve children, three vaccines taken together could alter immune systems and ultimately damage the brain. His findings landed in the British medical journal *The Lancet* and took the world by storm. But soon thereafter, his findings were declared fraudulent, as dozens of epidemiological studies found no merit to his work. His paper was retracted and the British medical authorities stripped him of his license to practice medicine.

But his legacy lives on in communities of people who still believe in his vaccine-autism link. Wakefield himself continues to support anti-vaccine rhetoric from here in the United States, creating fear among people who can benefit from life-saving vaccines. Among the initial leaders of the antivaccine movement have been celebrities with no medical degrees whatsoever, and popular bloggers with large online platforms. The science behind these vaccine-averse individuals isn't science at all. It's anecdotal evidence: "My son got the shot and then he wasn't the same." In Latin, there's an apt phrase for such fallacy in logic: *Post hoc, ergo propter hoc*. In English, "After this, therefore because of this." And in plainspeak: Event B follows Event A, so B must be the direct result of A.

Post hoc reasoning is the basis for many erroneous beliefs and even superstitions. An infinite number of events follow sequential patterns that appear to be cause and effect when in fact they are not related at all. For example, you forget your lucky charm and perform poorly on a test. You get a cold, so you drink more orange juice thinking the vitamin C will help, and you feel better a few days later. You get a flu shot and come down with a stuffy nose and sore throat within days, so you conclude it must have been the shot that made you sick. But sequences don't establish even a probability of causality any more than correlations do. Accidents and coincidences happen. When one thing happens after another, that doesn't mean the first thing caused the other.

Unfortunately, there's plenty of bad "evidence" going around the vaccine-autism debate to stir the pot of confusion. Antivaxxers, as they have been labeled, make their "scientific" case by cherry-picking a "peer-reviewed" paper that states what they believe, rather than looking at all the evidence before arriving at a conclusion. And if they did look at all the evidence, they'd have to find a way to reconcile the fact that there are more than one hundred articles that completely and utterly refute any causal link between the MMR vaccine and autism. For more than fifteen years, these papers, written by some of the world's best biomedical researchers in toxicology, neurology, immunology, microbiology, physiology, public health, and epidemiology, have been published in the top medical journals. The results have been repeated by independent researchers, and the statistical analyses are irrefutable.

But here's the other interesting thing: it's hard for us to change our beliefs. This is probably especially true when it comes to matters of life and health.

Motivated Reasoning

In 2014, a study came out that showed how stubborn we can be. It revealed that countering a big misperception can backfire. The study looked at people's concerns about the flu vaccine in particular; more than 4 in 10 Americans (43 percent) endorse the myth that the flu vaccine can infect you with the flu.[2] Some people believe it contains dangerous ingredients, such as mercury, formaldehyde, and antifreeze; that it can cause neurological disorders; that you don't need the vaccine if you've never had the flu; and that flu vaccines are a ploy for Big Pharma and doctors to profit, to name just a few of the myths.

Dartmouth researcher Brendan Nyhan, who led the study, noted that we tend to think that communication is a "silver bullet"—when someone corrects you using facts, such as the fact that a flu vaccine does not cause the flu, you'll then change your behavior and get a flu shot. But no, that actually isn't the case. Nyhan and his research partner, Jason Reifler of the University of Exeter, first created three groups by randomly dividing up 1,000 people. Then those people were asked how worried they were about serious side effects from vaccines. This allowed Nyhan and Reifler to identify those who were "very concerned" or "extremely concerned" about vaccines generally. Nearly a quarter of people (24 percent) overall met this criteria, and they were split up equally among the three groups.

Next, the researchers strategically dispensed information. They gave one group materials that detailed influenza's potential dangers. Another group got an explanation of how the flu vaccine cannot make you sick. And the third group received no information; they were left to stick to their own beliefs and assumptions. After the first two groups read the information, all the participants were asked more questions: How likely were they to get the flu vaccine this season? How safe did they think it was for most people? How accurate was it to say you can contract the flu from the flu vaccine?

The materials discrediting the myths of the flu vaccine did make a difference. Among the people most concerned about side effects, 70 percent of people in the group that didn't receive any information (the comparison group) thought the flu vaccine could give them the flu, compared with 51 percent who read the information debunking the myths. In those with the least concerns, 39 percent of the comparison group and 27 percent of those who read the myth-buster believed the fiction.

But here's where the social study got interesting. The debunking materials might have shifted people's perceptions of flu shots but not necessarily their intentions to get one. Less than half of those in the comparison group who worried about side effects said they planned to get the vaccine, which isn't surprising since they didn't read the materials. But only 28 percent of people with high concerns who read the flu facts said they *might* get one, as none of these "concerned" individuals had totally changed their mind. Saying that you might get the vaccine doesn't mean you will. In the words of Nyhan, "If you can't change their intentions, good luck changing their behavior." The study showed that even among those who were provided information about the dangers of the flu, the facts had no effect on their beliefs about vaccine safety or their intentions to vaccinate.

How did the researchers explain this odd behavior that defies logic and common sense? Clearly, if misperceptions of the facts support the antivaccination mentality, then invalidating those myths should increase people's willingness to vaccinate. But that didn't necessarily happen in this experiment, suggesting that misperceptions about vaccines "may be a reflection of less favorable attitudes toward vaccines rather than a cause." In other words, people are going to believe what they want to believe—and those beliefs will drive their behaviors.

Some experts in social psychology and cognitive science call this phenomenon "motivated reasoning." We make decisions based largely on emotions; it's our unconscious tendency to fit information to conclusions that suit some end or goal. Put another way, we essentially move the goalposts in our arguments to meet our needs and conclusions while ignoring contrary data, even if there's plenty of it. People who use motivated reasoning respond defensively to contrary evidence. They actively discredit such evidence or its source without logical or evidentiary justification. It's confirmation bias to the extreme.

Why do we defend obvious falsehoods? It can't be just to always feel as if we're right. Social scientists posit that our desire to avoid "cognitive dissonance," as they call it, drives motivated reasoning. In other words, self-delusion feels good.

Dan Kahan is a professor of law at Yale Law School. He explains a classic example of motivated reasoning by describing an experiment done in the 1950s when psychologists asked students from two Ivy League universities to watch a film that featured a set of controversial calls made by referees during a football game.[3] The game happened to be between teams from their respective schools. The students from each school were more likely to interpret the referees' calls as correct when they benefited their school's team than when they favored their rival. The psychologists concluded that the emotional stake the students had in affirming their loyalty to their respective institutions colored what they saw on the tape.

I love how American satirist H. L. Mencken put it: "The most common of all follies is to believe passionately in the palpably not true. It is the chief occupation of mankind." In *Brave New World*, Aldous Huxley wrote, "One believes things because one has been conditioned to believe them."

This can be harmful in health circles because it drives foolish ideas that spread over the internet, attracting new subscribers who just don't know how to distinguish between what's truth and what's less than the whole truth or utterly false. Claims that vaccines cause autism, that climate change is a hoax, and that AIDS is not caused by HIV are all examples of motivated reasoning.

In the Lucky Years, we'll need to reshape our context continually and adapt quickly to new data, especially the kind that should change our behaviors and ways of thinking. But right now, we see what we want to see. We think what we want to think. And we'll go to the end of the earth (even if we think it's flat and that the sun revolves around it) to protect our coveted beliefs.

So is there any point in countering all the mythology that lives in our society today so we can benefit more in the Lucky Years? Of course there is. You may not succeed in convincing every person, but, hopefully, you can tip the scales in favor of the reliable data so newcomers can absorb the facts first before being convinced of something else. First impressions count.

Surprisingly, in the flu vaccine study, people with low concerns about it were no more or less likely to get the vaccine after reading the corrective information. Nyhan brings up a good point: perhaps mentioning the myth to begin with may have negative effects. Earlier research has shown that reminding people of the myth can have the effect of validating it in their minds, creating an "illusion of truth" that may reinforce those falsehoods. Unfortunately, we in the scientific community don't know yet how to present data in ways that will reliably persuade people to change their minds.

The vaccine wars of today, stirred up most recently by outbreaks of vaccine-preventable diseases like whooping cough and measles, are nothing new. They are as old as vaccination itself. When Edward Jenner, a brilliant English country doctor, developed the vaccine for smallpox in 1796, he was both praised and mocked, lauded and feared. Religious authorities accused him of playing God, and even the equally bright economist Thomas Malthus lost sleep over the thought that vaccines would lead to unsustainable surges in the number of people on the planet. And when people first heard about getting an injection of foreign animal matter into their bodies, they were taken aback.[4] Jenner himself was the butt of jokes as cartoons emerged showing cows' horns shooting up from the heads of recently vaccinated people.

I'm a big proponent for vaccination among those who are eligible. Vaccines are not just for children hoping to avoid the ills of yesteryear like polio and chicken pox. When the scientific data clearly and overwhelmingly prove that a particular vaccine can reduce the risk of contracting a certain illness dramatically with few to no side effects, then we as a society should demand universal inoculation (the only exception being those who cannot be vaccinated due to certain disorders or because they are immune compromised). Much in the way we prevent our kids from suffering from measles and diphtheria, we can prevent adults from experiencing serious—and sometimes fatal—afflictions

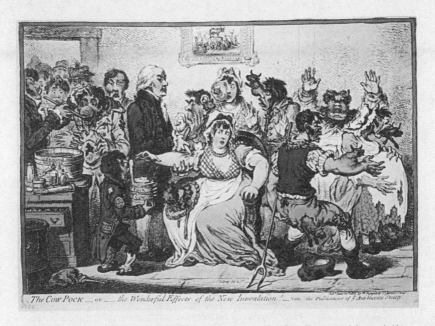

The Cow Pock _ or _ the Wonderful Effects of the New Inoculation ! _ vide the Publications of ye Anti Vaccine Society

In this cartoon, James Gillray drew a scene at the Smallpox and Inoculation Hospital at St. Pancras, showing Jenner's cowpox vaccine being administered to frightened young women, and cow parts emerging from the subjects' bodies. The cartoon was inspired by the controversy at the time over administering materials from animals to humans.

that nowadays have inexpensive and painless antidotes in the form of a vaccine. These include the human papilloma virus, influenza, pneumonia, and shingles. This mandate alone can likely put a big dent in our rates of communicable diseases later in life, and, as a result, bring health care costs down significantly.

The Nocebo Effect and the Limits of Nutritional Studies

In 2015, while attending the World Economic Forum in Davos, Switzerland, I found myself in an uncomfortable position while on a panel about nutrition called "Let Food Be Thy Medicine." I was once again reminded of the limits and pitfalls of our own belief systems.

The panel was intended to explore how our daily diet and dietary habits can become a cornerstone of health. I got the conversation started with statements that most people probably didn't want to hear. Nutrition is one of the thorniest topics in health; it tends to get underneath people's skins. Everyone has an opinion on the subject and there is so much conflicting data in this area that the noise becomes deafening.

One question I like to raise is what exactly *is* nutrition? How can we define it? For someone like me, who tells two or three people a week that I have nothing left to give them to extend their lives, let alone cure them, it's frustrating that we don't have reliable data from nutrition that show how to prevent disease and live longer through specific dietary protocols. If we did, then the pendulum wouldn't swing so wildly back and forth on what's considered "good" for us. Just reflect on what you've experienced in your own life. Most of us have learned to view eggs and other animal products like red meat as infrequent indulgences due to their fat and cholesterol content. Americans have been told to choose a low-fat diet rich in whole grains and complex carbohydrates. But in the fall of 2014, experts on the government's committee charged with setting dietary guidelines changed their tune. They acknowledged that there was "no appreciable relationship" between dietary cholesterol and blood cholesterol.[5] They also admitted that a low-fat diet may not be ideal.

What makes nutrition studies and their resulting policies so challenging is that they rely on observational examinations during which researchers follow large groups of people over long periods, keeping track of what they are eating and what the outcomes are. This is not, however, the best kind of science. They often base their findings on questionnaires in which people rely on their memories to recall their dietary and other choices. But think about that: if you're enrolled in a study and asked about how many times you raided the cookie jar or visited a fast-food restaurant in the past week or month, how honest and reliable can you be? Even the most rigorous observational studies can only produce results that show associations, not causation. In other words, such studies can suggest hypotheses (e.g., saturated fats are linked to heart disease), but fail to really prove anything (e.g., saturated fats *cause* heart disease).

So in the end, there really is no firm data in this department. Just a lot of generalized statements and anecdotal evidence: "I went on a gluten-free diet and felt amazing," "I went Paleo and lost forty pounds," "I cut out sugar and grew stronger nails and longer hair." While I think we all can agree that a diet high in processed sugars and fats won't do anyone good, it's hard to make scientifically proven conclusions about all the nuances of nutrition. I do have hope that one day we'll be able to conduct nutrition studies that can rule out all the variables and offer reliable recommendations. Even then, however, those recommendations may not be for everyone. That's why I'm a big believer in taking nutrition into your own hands and doing what the great medieval philosopher Maimonides suggested: try everything and see how certain foods and dietary protocols make you feel. Listen to your body and follow its signals. There may never be a right and wrong way to eat. Diet is contextual. Keep in mind that people have been eating various diets based on their cultures for thousands of years—diets that have sustained populations and allowed them to live good, long lives. Only in modern Western civilization do we incessantly search for the heroes and villains in our dietary habits and label them as such.

Although we have some evidence that a Mediterranean diet, for example, is associated with a reduced risk of death from heart disease and cancer, as well as a lower incidence of Parkinson's and Alzheimer's diseases, that's not to say other diets are therefore bad or increase the risk of these ailments. Some traditional populations in Africa, such as the Maasai people in Kenya and Tanzania, live primarily off raw milk and raw blood and occasional meat from cattle. And—surprise!—they have low incidence of the diseases typically attributed to a high-fat, high-cholesterol diet, such as heart disease and cancer. So how do we reconcile that fact in our modern arguments about the ills of meat, dairy, and not having a diverse diet?

The gluten debate is a particularly intriguing one. Countless people swear by a gluten-free diet, which avoids the foods in which the protein composite gluten is found: wheat, rye, barley, and other grains. Gluten is what gives bread its delicious chewiness. Gluten-free is a big industry. Sales of gluten-free products are estimated to hit $15 billion in 2016, and nearly a third of Americans try to avoid the ingredient. These people believe that gluten causes intestinal distress even in the absence of celiac disease, an autoimmune disorder triggered by gluten that affects only 1 percent of Americans. Celiac patients must avoid gluten, but why is everyone else jumping on this bandwagon? Is there really such a thing as non-celiac gluten sensitivity?

Peter Gibson of Monash University in Australia is one of the researchers who first documented non-celiac gluten sensitivity in a small study he published in 2011.[6] But after careful thinking, Gibson wasn't satisfied with his results. He wondered, as I would, how a compound so ubiquitous in any diet today could be cause for serious concern for so many people. So Gibson returned to the drawing board and upped the ante on his experiments. He took his next experiment to the extreme, which isn't something we normally see happen in nutrition studies. He attempted to validate—or invalidate—his previous finding.

What he did was clever.[7] He took 37 people who claimed to be gluten sensitive and had irritable bowel syndrome (IBS) and provided them with meals that eliminated ingredients associated with gastrointestinal distress in some people. These potential triggers included lactose (from milk products); certain preservatives like propionate, sulfites, and nitrites; and fermentable, poorly absorbed short-chain carbohydrates (technically known as fermentable oligo-di-monosaccharides and polyols, or FODMAPs). He also collected nine days' worth of urine and poop, presumably to ensure no one cheated. The individuals cycled through different diets—high-gluten, low-gluten, and no-gluten—but they didn't know which diet plan they were on at any given time. And guess what: all of the diets—even the gluten-free diet—allegedly caused gas, bloating, pain, and nausea to a similar degree. It didn't matter if the diet contained gluten. In the words of Gibson: "In contrast to our first study . . . we could find absolutely no specific response to gluten."[8]

Although this was also a small study, another larger one published later on confirmed the findings.

How do we explain this unexpected result? This is where the science gets interesting. It could be that people *expected* to feel worse on the study's diets, so they did—a phenomenon called the "nocebo" effect, a wordplay on the placebo effect. After all, they did have to pay close attention to how their tummies felt, which alone might entail some psychosomatic response. Moreover, it's been suggested that gluten may be the wrong villain and that these other potential triggers, especially the FODMAPs, are to blame. These ingredients often travel with gluten. It may in fact be the carbohydrate component rather than the gluten part of the wheat that is causing symptoms. Other constituents of wheat might also be problematic for some people. That said, it still doesn't explain why people in the study reacted negatively to diets that were free of all dietary triggers. Which is why sweeping, absolute statements like "Gluten is always bad" or "Organic is always good" miss the point, especially when it comes to preventing illnesses. The difference between good and bad revolves around individual context; what is right for each person is a highly individualized matter, especially in light of the fact that too much of the science about nutrition does not always hold up.

I'm all for prevention. It's the best way today to avoid the illnesses that can take our lives prematurely, especially cancer. But we can't make blanket statements about the superior power of prevention through dietary strategies alone, to the exclusion of other therapies. A new buzzword has crept into the lay vernacular: *lifestyle medicine*. This term refers to using basic lifestyle interventions—nutrition, exercise, supplementation, stress management—to prevent and sometimes even treat disease rather than pharmaceutical drugs to do so. But here's the thing: this conversation gets corrupted by the same black-and-white thinking that plagues many other areas of health. There are lots of ways to reach a goal, and those ways should be distinct to each individual.

The Hazards of Broad, Sweeping Statements

Given my views on this subject, you can imagine my reaction on that World Economic Forum panel when my colleague Dean Ornish, a physician and researcher based in San Francisco who is focused on preventive medicine mostly through diet, said bluntly: "Drugs and surgery don't work nearly as well as we once thought."[9] He was speaking within the context of treating heart patients, but then went on to say more specifically that diabetes and heart disease drugs don't work in certain situations, and he referred to one of his own studies that concluded "intensive lifestyle interventions" can positively affect the progression of early-stage prostate cancer. I immediately protested against his broad assertions, which frankly made me look terrible—like the bad guy who prefers drugs from Big Pharma. But Ornish's 2005 study shows how declaratory statements, especially from a small study such as this one, can be misleading and cause confusion.

I should preface this story with the fact that Ornish's original claim to fame was the reversal of heart disease through lifestyle changes. But cancer is an entirely different animal. So when he broached my subject area in our panel discussion, my ears pricked up. The purpose of Ornish's twelve-month study was to examine the impact of changes in diet and lifestyle to men with early-stage, low-grade prostate cancer.[10] All of the 93 men in the experiment had chosen not to undergo an active treatment. Due to the low-risk nature of their prostate cancer, they opted for a "watchful waiting" (which is now called "active surveillance") approach instead of conventional treatment such as surgery, drugs, and/or radiation. Active surveillance, which is now routine for early-stage prostate cancers, means following the disease and doing repeat biopsies on a regular basis, and only treating the disease if it progresses.

The men were randomly assigned either to an experimental group that was asked to make comprehensive lifestyle changes or to a "usual care" control group. "Usual care" meant following their doctor's advice in terms of general lifestyle changes. However, the study was designed to decrease the likelihood that control group patients would make diet and lifestyle changes comparable to those of the experimental group, thereby making the results difficult to interpret. There were 44 men in the experimental group and 49 men in the control. The actual lifestyle intervention taken by the 44 men was the following:

- vegan diet supplemented with soy (1 daily serving of tofu plus 58 grams of a fortified soy protein powdered beverage)
- fish oil (3 grams daily)
- vitamin E (400 IU daily)
- selenium (200 micrograms daily)
- vitamin C (2 grams daily)
- moderate aerobic exercise (walking 30 minutes 6 days weekly)
- stress-management techniques (gentle yoga-based stretching, breathing, meditation, imagery, and progressive relaxation for a total of 60 minutes daily)
- participation in a weekly 1-hour support group to enhance adherence to the intervention

The diet of the intervention group was predominantly fruits, vegetables, whole grains (complex carbohydrates), legumes, and soy products. It also was low in simple carbohydrates and included approximately 10 percent of its calories from fat.

The results looked at a common marker in evaluating the progression of prostate cancer: PSA, prostate-specific antigen, a protein produced by prostate gland cells. Elevated levels of PSA in the blood can signal changes in the prostate, including prostate cancer. Here's what Ornish's experiment found: the serum PSA decreased an average of 0.25 ng/ml, or 4 percent of the baseline average in the experimental group. But in the control group PSA levels increased an average of 0.38 ng/ml or 6 percent of the baseline average. Now, what does this really mean? Despite the slight "increase" and "decrease," the change was not clinically significant in medical terms. And here's the kicker: a change in PSA doesn't mean you change the disease or the disease outcome at all. Ornish published no follow-up to his study, so we have no idea what happened to these men. We don't know if they lived longer or not. We also don't know if the cancer progressed more or less in the lifestyle group.

Put another way, disease wasn't measured in this experiment—only the PSA. My guess is the PSA was lowered due to the estrogenic effects of the dietary soy; soy notoriously reduces PSA in men but has no bearing on the actual cancer. This same problem crops up in studies done on the effects of saw palmetto, a popular over-the-counter herbal remedy touted to lower PSA. It does, but artificially, by lowering testosterone. It doesn't touch the cancer! A change to one marker, in these cases a lower PSA, may not be meaningful. And weight loss may have been a huge factor, if not the main game changer. The lifestyle group participants lost an average of 10 pounds on the study.

And yet bold, sweeping statements were made in the media about Ornish's results: "Lifestyle Changes May Slow Prostate Cancer Progression" and "Improving Diet, Lifestyle Slows Prostate Cancer." The other weird thing about the Ornish paper, published in the *Journal of Urology*, is that it reported only the average PSA of each group, which is meaningless when managing patients on an individual basis. One outlier in a small study, for example, can move the entire number and thereby alter the results dramatically. I know of no other cancer studies that report results like that. Usually the number reported is the percentage of patients who have a PR (partial response), meaning greater than 50 percent shrinkage of a tumor or 50 percent lowering of PSA.

I get scared when anyone makes broad statements like "Lifestyle can reverse cancer," but it's especially alarming when these come from people who are considered leading experts. While I can concede that lifestyle may in fact impact cancer outcomes, there is currently no hard evidence of this. And let me push the envelope a little further by asking the question: Was this study looking at lifestyle factors? Who defines "lifestyle"? I count five medications, in the form of vitamins and supplements, taken by the experimental group. Even more worrisome is that vitamin E was used, and we now have solid evidence from large-scale studies clearly showing that vitamin E supplementation can *increase* the incidence of prostate cancer. One multicenter study led by Fred Hutchinson Cancer Research Center has found that high-dose supplementation with both the trace element selenium and vitamin E increases the risk of high-grade prostate cancer.[11] These findings, published in 2014 in the *Journal of the National Cancer Institute*, are based on data from the Selenium and Vitamin E Cancer Prevention Trial, or SELECT, a well-designed trial conducted by the SWOG cancer research cooperative group that involved more than 35,000 men. The scientists behind the study wanted to determine whether taking high-dose vitamin E (400 IU/day) and/or selenium (200 mcg/day) supplements could protect men from prostate cancer.

The trial began in 2001 and was supposed to last twelve years. But it was halted early, in 2008, because it found no protective effect from selenium, and there was a hint that vitamin E increased risk. Even though the use of the study supplements ended, the researchers continued to follow the men. After an additional two years, those who had taken vitamin E had a statistically significant 17 percent increased risk of prostate cancer.

Let's take a look at one more study, this one more recent and which really hit a nerve in my medical community after it was published in *Science*. The headline from Johns Hopkins University media department said it all: "Bad Luck of Random Mutations Plays Predominant Role in Cancer, Study Shows."[12]

Up in Smoke

In early 2015, during the holiday lull around New Year's, a study by mathematician Cristian Tomasetti and cancer geneticist Bert Vogelstein of Johns Hopkins suggested "bad luck"—random mutations accumulating in healthy stem cells—could explain about two-thirds of cancers.[13] In other words, the media reported, cancer occurs mostly by chance—arbitrary, unexplained mutations lead to most cancers rather than the risks conferred by environmental and genetic factors combined (so go ahead and keep eating your potato chips, smoking, and avoiding exercise). They also seemed to suggest, based on their findings, that some cancers could not be prevented and that detecting them early was key to combating them. It didn't take long for there to be a backlash against the implied message. Tomasetti and Vogelstein were accused of focusing on rare cancers while leaving out several common cancers that indeed are largely preventable. The International Agency for Research on Cancer, the cancer arm of the World Health Organization, published a press release stating it "strongly disagrees" with the report.

To arrive at their conclusion, Tomasetti and Vogelstein used a statistical model they developed based on known rates of cell division in thirty-one types of tissue. Stem cells were their main focal point. As a reminder, these are the small, specialized "mothership" cells in each organ or tissue that divide to replace cells that die or wear out. Only in recent years have researchers been able to conduct these kinds of studies due to advances in the understanding of stem-cell biology. Cells that divide must make copies of their DNA, and errors in this delicate process, as you know by now, can spark the uncontrolled growth that leads to cancer.

The researchers sought to answer the following: Do higher rates of stem-cell division up the risk of cancer simply by providing more room for error? More chances for mistakes? Dr. Vogelstein, who is one of Hopkins's most prolific and esteemed cancer researchers, said the question of what causes cancer had bothered him for decades, ever since he was a young intern and one of his first patients was an impressionable four-year-old girl with leukemia. Like any distraught parents with a sick child, hers wanted to know what had brought on the disease. He didn't know and couldn't provide a reasonable, acceptable answer. He'd be asked this same troubling question from patients and their families repeatedly, particularly from parents of children with cancer. Parents of children who die of cancer can be somewhat comforted knowing that it might have happened by chance, that there was nothing they could have done, and that it didn't come from them. But cancer in children might work differently than cancer in adults. Clearly, children haven't had a lifetime to accumulate risk factors for genetic mutations that can lead to cancer. So their cancer's narrative is probably not the same as that for most adults.

This wasn't the first time scientists had discovered different cancer rates in different tissues. After all, you rarely hear about someone getting ear cancer or heart cancer. Cancers of the small intestine's lining are three times less common than brain tumors, even though the cells that line the small intestine are exposed to much higher levels of environmental toxins that can cause cellular mutations than are cells within the brain, which are largely protected by the blood-brain barrier. So what explains this discrepancy?

More than one hundred years ago it was observed that some tissues are far more susceptible to developing cancer than others. But we didn't know why and we couldn't give a reason for it. That observation motivated Tomasetti and Vogelstein to dig a little deeper and try to understand why, for example, the lifetime risk for cancer in the large intestine is 24 times higher than in the small intestine. What they found is that the large intestine houses more stem cells than the small intestine. Moreover, the large intestine's stem cells divide four times more frequently than do the stem cells in the small intestine. This relationship between rates of stem-cell division and risk of cancer was also seen in many other tissues. Unfortunately, their analysis didn't include two of the most common types of cancer—breast and prostate—because there wasn't enough information on rates of stem-cell division in those tissues, an omission that was criticized by others upon their reporting.

Interestingly, they noted that some cancers, such as those of the lung and skin, develop more often than would be expected from their rates of stem-cell division. But this makes sense when you consider the impact of environmental forces in the risk of those diseases, namely smoking and UV exposure from the sun, respectively. Other cancers found to be more common than expected given their stem-cell division rates were linked to genes that cause cancer, which again helps explain that surprising difference. Dr. Tomasetti used an apt analogy when he described his results in an addendum to the original news release from Hopkins that created such a stir: Think of your risk of a car accident. In general, the more you drive or the longer the trip, the higher the odds of a crash. But other forces are also at play that add to and/or compound the risk, namely environmental ones like awful weather and poor roads (bad habits), as well as defects in the car itself (bad genes). The researchers finally got their message right when they stated the following:

> Some risk factors may be outside of our control, but others are not. The fact that much of the risk of traveling by car is due simply to the trip distance doesn't mean that accidents cannot be prevented. Distance is one factor, but even if the distance of a trip cannot be changed, traveling can be made safer by driving well-maintained vehicles, using safety devices, such as seatbelts and airbags, and choosing a particular route. Controlling the risk of accidents associated with bad cars and bad roads prevents accidents and reduces overall risk.
>
> In the same way, we can prevent many cancers. Like car accidents, cancer is caused by a combination of factors—random DNA changes made during stem cell divisions that are not within our control, environmental exposures and inherited gene mutations. As a result, there are many opportunities for cancer prevention . . . by eliminating environmental factors and by changing lifestyles.[14]

This addendum, which also underscored the importance of detecting and treating cancer early to prevent death, was published within days of the original news release. But I'm not sure many people read it or got the message through those same journalists who misinterpreted the original report.

Where critics and journalists went wrong in their analysis of the study was that Tomasetti and Vogelstein weren't suggesting that two-thirds of all cancers are due to chance. They were showing that two-thirds of *the variation in cancer rates in different tissues* could be explained by random bad luck. Put another way, some tissues are more vulnerable to cancer than others, and mutations piling up in stem cells can explain two-thirds of that variability. A subtle but very important distinction, one that many of the journalists reporting on the study missed, hence the misleading headlines suggesting most cancer is random and not influenced by heredity or lifestyle choices.

To say that a "bad luck" component explains a far greater number of cancers than do hereditary and environmental factors is doing a disservice to public health, especially since the lay public doesn't have the expertise to tease out the nuances and finer details of this complex study and its even more complex conclusions. And what really infuriates me, as someone who stares cancer in the face daily, is that people have begun to take advantage of this inaccuracy for profit. My dear friend Esther Dyson, a prominent journalist and technology leader whose focus lately, ironically, has been none other than improving efficacy in health care, became the target of predatory practices in health care. She forwarded the sales pitch in a message to me with the following remark: "This wretched Hopkins study is now being used by sleazy marketers." Indeed, it was:

Hi Esther,

I am writing to bring your attention to new research from Johns Hopkins, which demonstrates that ⅔ of cancers are due to bad luck, thus making it difficult to avoid solely through lifestyle modifications (e.g., not smoking, diet, etc.). Therefore, the best prevention remains intensive surveillance. That's why we provide the most comprehensive preventive physical possible including upgraded imaging and laboratory screening. . . . It is the same program of care as received by the President of the United States, and a 2011 study in the *Journal of the American Medical Association* (*JAMA*) has already proven that Presidents live much longer than expected. We would like to ensure that you have the same opportunity for good health and longevity. Therefore, we are expanding our membership capability with the addition of other highly qualified physicians who specialize in preventive medicine.

We would be glad to welcome you as a member of our program . . .

In a word: unbelievable. I wonder how many other marketers sold people on expensive services they probably don't need, reinforcing their desire to leave their health in the hands of others rather than make their own daily choices. Don't get me wrong: there's always a place for preventive screenings and, sometimes, "intensive surveillance," but we cannot ignore the power of prevention through a combination of lifestyle habits and other therapies. Just as cancer is likely a result of a constellation of forces—genetic, environmental, behavioral—our efforts to prevent it should take all those factors into account. And we can't forget one of the most powerful forces of all underlying most diseases, cancer included: inflammation. This word was surprisingly left out of the entire dialogue about the Hopkins study, including the authors themselves and the critics who threw tomatoes.

Where There's Smoke, There's Fire

Inflammation is a word and a concept that has gained a lot of notoriety in the past decade. It's been written about daily in health media, for it seems to have a relationship to virtually all manner of chronic and degenerative disease. Whether it's the tenderness of a sore throat, the redness that appears after a cut, or the achiness of an arthritic joint, most of us understand that when the body experiences an insult or injury, its natural response is to create swelling and pain, hallmarks of the inflammatory process. But inflammation isn't necessarily bad. It's a symptom of the body's defense mechanisms against something it identifies and responds to as potentially harmful. When the body is tending to an open wound, harmful virus or bacteria, toxins, or sprained ankle, the inflammatory process is ultimately helping it to survive.

The problem with inflammation, and the source of its negative reputation today, is that it can get out of control. A fire hose turned on momentarily to douse nearby flames is one thing, but leave that hose on indefinitely and you've got another problem on your hands soon enough. And that's the case with inflammation gone awry. It's intended to be a spot treatment, not an ongoing process. If the body is constantly under assault by exposure to irritants, the inflammatory response stays on. This creates an imbalance in your system that has negative effects on your health as it spreads to every part of the body through the bloodstream; hence, we have the ability to detect this kind of widespread inflammation through blood tests—notably by looking for markers such as C-reactive protein. It can even disrupt the immune system and lead to chronic problems and/or disease.

Inflammation may not seem related to many conditions and afflictions, especially cancer, but volumes of international research prove just how damaging chronic inflammation can be to the body. Certain kinds of inflammation have been linked to most degenerative diseases, including heart disease, Alzheimer's disease, autoimmune diseases, diabetes, and cancer. It's also associated with accelerated aging and premature death. At the center of inflammation is the concept of oxidative stress, which, in a rudimentary sense, is like a biological type of corrosion that takes place in our organs and tissues. It can damage our cells' structures and functionality, stiffen blood vessels, tinker with hormonal switches, and even target DNA, precipitating mutations and mistakes in translation when DNA is used to make various proteins necessary for the body's operations. Oxidation is actually normal. It happens everywhere in nature, including our bodies. When we digest food, for example, and the body turns it into energy, oxidation is a natural part of the process. But, like inflammation, oxidation becomes a problem when unchecked.

So what does inflammation have to do with the Hopkins study? The road to cancer in any given tissue involves inflammation, which has been correlated with the development of cancer for a long time. In fact, you can't have a conversation about cancer without talking about inflammation. When you hear that certain infections, such as the human papillomavirus (HPV) or the hepatitis B and hepatitis C viruses, can lead to cancer, much of the reason is rooted in inflammation. Epidemiological studies estimate that nearly 15 percent of the worldwide cancer incidence is associated with microbial infection.[15] Why? These infections cause chronic irritation in the body and keep the immune system "on edge," and this causes ongoing inflammation that predisposes cells to cancer. The same can be said for anything that continually irritates the body and its immune system: high blood sugar, diabetes, obesity, tobacco use.

The actual process by which chronic inflammation results in cancerous cells is exceedingly complex, and it may be different depending on which type of cell we're talking about and which type of cancer. But the overall picture is an important one to remember: when the body experiences chronic inflammation, something isn't right and the body's attempt to bring things back into balance can be sabotaged by that persistent inflammation, leaving cells—and their inherent DNA— vulnerable.

Cells possess innate mechanisms to prevent rampant, uncontrolled proliferation or the accumulation of DNA mutations (recall the DNA mismatch repair system I described earlier). In the face of DNA damage or the hint of a crazy cell activating tumor growth, cells will either repair their DNA and prevent mutations or the deranged cells will self-destruct. However, when you have an infection or there's other injury to tissue that leads to inflammation, massive cell death is likely a step in the path to recovery. When a tissue loses such a large number of cells at once, those lost cells must be replaced to keep the tissue functioning, and stem cells often self-renew and divide to fill the gap. So inflammation is used to defend the body, and it's used to initiate the healing process and repair tissue. But it's also sending proliferative signals to cells that have the potential to become cancerous.

When the Hopkins study suggested that cancer is often due to "bad luck of random mutations," the researchers left this important cascade of events out of the narrative. What if you're an overweight smoker who is diagnosed with pelvic bone cancer, a super-rare cancer? Anyone's lifetime risk of getting this cancer is a mere 0.003 percent; consider that against the lifetime risk for each of us of being diagnosed with lung cancer, which is 6.9 percent. So you might think you were somewhat lucky in that you didn't get lung cancer as a smoker, but instead you developed this other cancer by the hand of "bad luck." But let's connect the dots: smoking kept your body continually fighting that nasty habit's negative biological effects. And we know that tobacco and all of its insidious ingredients don't just affect the lungs in a vacuum. Tobacco affects virtually every cell and system in the body. It's not a far stretch of the imagination to see how tobacco can trigger genetic mutations that manifest in a cancer anywhere in the body, perhaps in a place where you're already genetically susceptible to cancer. Maybe you've got good genes to protect you from lung cancer, but not so much for bone cancer. We all know people who smoke long past their eightieth birthday and die of something other than lung cancer, or the fellow who gorges on fatty, sugary foods daily but never gets diabetes. These people aren't necessarily "lucky"; no doubt their habits are fanning flames of inflammation in their body that will manifest in other, less obvious ailments or in conditions that do not at first glance seem to be related directly to their poor lifestyle choices. But we cannot chalk it all up to purely bad luck.

Indeed, life is a genetic gamble to a large degree. We have to play the cards dealt us, but we can stack the odds in our favor by controlling our exposure to environmental and lifestyle factors (e.g., not smoking, eating well, getting our exercise, using technologies to stay on top of our health status, etc.). Suggesting cancer is mostly due to bad luck dilutes the important message that some risk can be modified by behavior. My guess is that future studies and technologies will be able to tell us that even the most elusive, rare types of cancer that seem to be due to bad luck can actually be influenced by our environment and lifestyle. And knowing that cancer is preventable and can be impacted by behavior is, to me, empowering.

Most Medical Studies Are Wrong

Regrettably, most medical studies are wrong; they are biased and flawed, each in its own unique way. By some estimates, on average only 3,000 of 50,000 new journal articles published every year are sufficiently well designed and relevant to inform patient care.[16] That's 6 percent. A whopping 94 percent of studies published do not carry significant enough valid data to warrant a change in how doctors treat patients, nor will their findings impact patient outcomes. Richard Horton, the current editor in chief of *The Lancet*, has been critical of the reliability in published research despite the fact that he's at the helm of one of the most well-respected medical journals in the world. In a 2015 comment published in his journal, he went so far as to say, "The case against science is straightforward: much of the scientific literature, perhaps half, may simply be untrue. Afflicted by studies with small sample sizes, tiny effects, invalid exploratory analyses, and flagrant conflicts of interest, together with an obsession for pursuing fashionable trends of dubious importance, science has taken a turn towards darkness." [17]

Other leading physicians and researchers have echoed these critical sentiments, including Marcia Angell, a Harvard doctor and former editor in chief of the *New England Journal of Medicine*. It doesn't help that studies that appear to be well done have their competition that shows wildly different outcomes. One study will have a conclusion that's totally opposite to another study's bottom line. Look no further than the research on foods that cause or prevent cancer to appreciate this disconnect. The truth is somewhere in the totality of the research, but unfortunately the media reports on every study in isolation underneath contradicting headlines. [18]

In 2013, a couple of researchers from Harvard and Stanford teamed up to randomly select fifty ingredients from recipes in *The Boston Cooking-School Cook Book*, then searched PubMed to see which of the ingredients had been linked with either increasing or decreasing the risk of cancer. [19] They identified forty, including staples like bread, potatoes, tomatoes, wine, tea, milk, eggs, coffee, butter, beef, and corn—foods that we all have heard both positive and negative things about. One of the researchers, John Ioannidis of Stanford, had already delved into this world more than ten years ago when he published "Why Most Published Research Findings Are False," which became one of the most cited papers in *PLOS Medicine*. [20] His latest investigations culminated in his 2013 paper showing that, for the most part, pretty much everything we eat both causes and prevents cancer. And when it comes to things like milk, eggs, bread, and butter, you can find just as many studies that support their health benefits as their cancer-causing risks.

Scientists can have difficulty getting their papers accepted into prestigious journals. In a world of "publish or perish," this has created a market for bottom-feeding journals with impressive-sounding names but absolutely no standards. The number of published medical studies has skyrocketed accordingly, with a 300 percent increase over the last twenty-five years.[21] And the so-called open-access model, which allows anyone to access certain journals freely online without paying a fee, has given rise to a slew of online publishers, many of which are unscrupulous and exist only to make money off the authors who pay to have their papers published. The authors' reports (and research results) are not filtered or challenged by the scientific rigors of traditionally published peer-reviewed journals that maintain high-quality standards in accepting papers and making them available to the research community. Most respectable studies involve several leading experts and many months of editorial and scientific scrutiny, and back and forth discourse, before they are published. With some rare exceptions, anything can get published relatively quickly by these open-access journals regardless of the quality and validity of the research methods, data, and conclusions. In 2011, the number of predatory publishers was only 18; by 2014, that number had ballooned to 477.[22] What all this really means is that information not driven by real data is seeping into the medical literature, and mainstream media journalists will often base their articles and arguments on these shoddy papers that should never have made it to publication. The need for skepticism has never been greater.

The lesson: seek multiple sources that arrive at the same answer. Until we have better curators of medical wisdom in our country for the benefit of all, each one of us must play the curator role in our individual lives.

In my first book, I condemned vitamin D supplementation alongside taking vitamins in general. At the time, millions of Americans had been told they were deficient in vitamin D and were taking megadoses of it in a bid to bring their levels up to what was considered "normal."

To most people, this seemed like an obvious problem to remedy, for previous research claimed that vitamin D deficiency in adults could cause fractures, falls, functional limitations, cancer, diabetes, cardio-vascular disease, depression, and higher risk of death in general. We get vitamin D through certain foods but mostly through UV exposure to the sunlight, which stimulates a reaction in the skin to produce this important hormone that's involved with a multitude of physiological functions. But given our use of sunscreen today and living at high lati-tudes, the thinking went, we probably weren't getting enough. Really? The body is much cleverer than that. It always has been.

Some advertising for the supplement went so far as to suggest that vitamin D could alleviate obesity, autoimmune disease, insomnia, and even autism. The jig was up following more research and meta-analyses of research to determine what should be considered "normal." The original definition was quite arbitrary and not many people, if any, who were deemed below "normal" were getting diagnosed with rickets, the soft-bone disease associated with a true deficiency. Yet so many blanket statements had been made about the benefits of vitamin D that people who hadn't even gotten their levels tested were taking it. New brands of vitamin D supplements flooded the market.

In the past few years, the whole idea of there being a widespread vitamin D deficiency and a need to test vitamin D levels, let alone supplement, has been called into question. Two new studies emerged in late 2013 that added to the growing body of evidence against the so-called sunshine vitamin. In one, a large review by Philippe Autier and colleagues at the International Prevention Research Institute in Lyon, France, it was found that taking supplemental vitamin D has no effect on a spectrum of diseases and conditions, from osteoporosis and bone diseases to heart disease, weight gain, multiple sclerosis, depression and other mood disorders, and metabolic disorders such as diabetes.[23] After looking at more than 450 studies, Autier and his colleagues con-cluded: "The absence of an effect of vitamin D supplementation on disease occurrence, severity, and clinical course leads to the hypothesis that variations [in vitamin D levels] would essentially be a result, and not a cause, of ill health." Put another way, we've had the cause and effect backward. Low vitamin D is the *result* of poor health—not the cause. The study stated: "Associations between 25(OH)D and health disorders . . . are not causal. Low 25(OH)D [vitamin D] could be the result of inflammatory processes involved in disease." In other words, low vitamin D levels could very well be signs of inflammation in the body, and correcting the alleged "low" vitamin D is just addressing a symptom—not a root cause of disease causing the inflammation.

Although Autier and his team didn't look at the biggest alleged benefit of vitamin D—protection against bone fractures—we have plenty of other studies to turn to and see that indeed, vitamin D doesn't help. We've long heard that vitamin D is associated with bone health, but it turns out that you can't get that benefit from a pill. As an aside, vitamin D isn't found in breast milk, likely because Mother Nature intended babies to get a little sunlight into their day. Maybe we're not supposed to consume vitamin D; we've evolved to make it in our skin using safe levels of UV rays that won't increase risk for skin cancer. In fact, in the same issue of *The Lancet* where Autier's study landed, a study done by Ian Reid and colleagues at the University of Auckland evaluated the vitamin D–bone health question.[24] They evaluated 23 studies with 4,082 participants, all designed to see if supplemental vitamin D improves bone density. And they arrived at the same conclusion: "Continuing widespread use of vitamin D for osteoporosis prevention in community-dwelling adults without specific risk factors for vitamin D deficiency seems to be inappropriate." To put it bluntly, vitamin D supplements are a waste of money. The whole notion that "more is better" needs to be dropped. We may want to do more in some areas of our lives, but this clearly shouldn't be one of them.

After another new report was published in the *Annals of Internal Medicine*, the US Preventive Services Task Force issued a statement in early 2015 saying that routine screening of asymptomatic patients for vitamin D deficiency was not necessary.[25] They cited what the *Annals* report found: there simply wasn't enough evidence to support the benefits or harms of screening for vitamin D deficiency.

Those who've followed my advice or read my previous writings know that I have no problem with people taking vitamins and supplements to address a true deficiency or condition, such as pregnancy. My frustration with the vitamin industry is actually less targeted at low-dose multivitamins and more geared to the megadose and stand-alone products that doctors recommend to patients without valid data to support their use, leaving many people confused and wasting money. Fish oil, for example, is the third most widely used dietary supplement, after vitamins and minerals. Many Americans—at least 10 percent by some estimates— take fish oil regularly in the belief that the omega-3 fatty acids in these supplements protect their heart.[26] But once again, the data doesn't speak this wisdom. The vast majority of clinical trials haven't found any conclusive evidence that fish oil supplements lower the risk of heart attack and stroke. Dozens of rigorous studies, most of which examined whether fish oil could prevent cardiovascular events in people who are at high risk, were published between 2005 and 2012 in the world's top medical journals.[27] These studies looked at people who were at high risk for heart problems, such as those with high cholesterol, high blood pressure, type 2 diabetes, or a history of heart disease. In all but two of these studies fish oil showed no benefit compared with a placebo.

Theoretically, it's reasonable to think that fish oil improves cardiovascular health. After all, most of these supplements contain two megastar omega-3 fatty acids—eicosapentaenoic acid (EPA) and docosahexaenoic acid (DHA). These fatty acids have been shown to reduce inflammation and have a blood-thinning effect, both of which factor into risk for cardiovascular events. The FDA has even approved at least three fish oil supplements that require a prescription; they are marketed for the treatment of high triglycerides (blood fats), a risk factor for heart disease. Despite the touted benefits of omega-3 fatty acids, they have not been observed in most large clinical trials. Only a change in a single lab test has been noted, which is quite meaningless.

The praise for fish oil began in the 1970s when the Danish scientists Drs. Hans Olaf Bang and Jorn Dyerberg noticed that Inuits living in northern Greenland enjoyed unusually low rates of cardiovascular disease. They credited this phenomenon to the Inuits' diet of omega-3-rich fats found in fish, seal, and whale blubber. But George Fodor, a cardiologist at the University of Ottawa, later pointed out the flaws in a lot of this early research, reckoning that the rate of heart disease among the Inuits was sorely underestimated. Fish oil supplements retained their halo effect, however, and this persists today.

Several studies that commenced in the 1990s also buoyed the case for fish oil. One study from Italy that was met with much fanfare, for example, found that heart attack survivors who were given a gram of fish oil daily had lower death rates compared with patients taking vitamin E.[28] These findings, published in 2002, motivated organizations like the American Heart Association to recommend fish oil supplements to people with heart conditions. But soon enough, people who didn't have any heart conditions or even risk factors for cardiovascular disease followed in a precautionary move.

No real benefit has been shown in recent studies, either, including one that involved the same Italian researcher who published those positive outcomes with fish oil more than a decade earlier. This study, featured in the *New England Journal of Medicine* in 2013, involved a clinical trial of 12,000 people and found that a daily gram of fish oil did not lower the death rate from heart attacks and strokes in people with atherosclerosis.[29] Atherosclerosis is a disease characterized by a buildup of fats, cholesterol, and other substances (collectively called plaques) in and on your artery walls. I should add that the early fish oil studies occurred in an era when cardiovascular disease was treated differently than it is today. Now we have powerful drugs at our disposal that can treat heart disease more effectively. Most of the cardiologists I know tell their patients to skip fish oil supplements and instead eat fatty fish at least twice a week. After all, fish contains an assortment of nutrients other than EPA and DHA. But many general practitioners will indeed recommend fish oil to their patients, as well as take it themselves despite the lack of incontrovertible data. Which highlights the fact that doctors don't always know what's right and want more research to be conducted to confirm or refute their thinking. That will happen in the Lucky Years.

One of the most common questions I get now is "My doctor told me to take X. What do I do?" The answer is simple: Ask your doctor "Why, and based on what data?" That's the conversation we all should be having, rather than reducing every health topic down to "This is categorically good" and "That is always bad." And I love it when I hear people say to me, "Thanks for explaining," as they let out a sigh of relief. I want people on as few drugs and supplements as possible, but at the same time I want people to employ the power of modern technologies—and medicines—whenever appropriate so that they may realize the ultimate goal: to take control of their health for a quality, long life.

The ultimate lesson here is to watch out for absolute, declaratory statements made by both media and experts alike, especially when they are taken out of context: "Reverse heart disease with this diet" . . . "Ax acne using this ingredient" . . . "Drink this smoothie to lose up to ten pounds a week" . . . "Look ten years younger by doing/taking the following" . . . "X will kill you" . . . "Y will make you fat" . . . "And Z will cure you . . ." Remember the three statements at the beginning of this chapter? Those are the kind of absolute announcements I'm talking about, and the answer to my pop quiz, if you hadn't already guessed, is that none of them is debatable; they're all false. Data is everywhere today, some of it sound but much of it questionable or in need of more study and explanation. Know where your data is coming from. Ask who, what, where, when, and *why*. If you learn how to look for reliable data, it will help you determine what is truly "best" for you.

CHAPTER 7

A Body in Motion Tends to Stay Lucky

The One Supplement You're Not Getting Enough Of

Lack of activity destroys the good condition of every human being, while movement and methodical physical exercise save it and preserve it.

—Plato

For centuries, we've known that exercise does a body good, even if the underlying scientific explanations were unknown or unclear. In the past decade, however, we've made huge strides in deciphering the extraordinary relationship between physical fitness and total health. This has been made possible by the latest technology and recent novel collaborations among various fields of science and medicine. The latest research has allowed us to measure, analyze, and understand biologically what happens when we flex our muscles, take a brisk walk, join a group fitness class, pedal a bicycle, pick up heavy boxes, or train for an athletic event.

We have been active animals in constant pursuit of survival since the birth of humankind. In fact, our genetic makeup requires and *expects* our bodies to be physically challenged via regular exercise. But as we are well aware, only a small percentage of us cater to our body's need to move frequently. Modern technology has its benefits, but it also has its drawbacks when it facilitates sitting all day. Most everything we need can be obtained without having to exert much effort, much less get off our butts. We didn't evolve over the past millions of years to thrive in a sitting position, and that fact has played into the rates of chronic illnesses that can be associated with being sedentary, such as diabetes and heart disease ("sitting diseases").

If we could go back in time to observe how ancient cultures took to sitting, we'd notice that many sat upright on floors in the cross-legged position, kneeled, or sat with "tent knees" with their buttocks and feet on the ground, knees bent. These positions require balance and coordination, as well as strength in the legs, glutes, and back. Now we use chairs and couches that have the unfortunate effect of putting the body in positions that are not ideal for its natural mechanics and circulation.

Nearly 80 percent of adult Americans do not get the recommended amounts of exercise each week.[1] A 2012 study led by Harvard researchers and published in *The Lancet* determined that inactivity is tied to more than 5 million deaths worldwide—more than those caused by smoking![2] A survey of nearly thirty thousand women in the United States done the following year found that those who sat nine or more hours a day were more likely to be depressed than those who sat fewer than six hours a day.[3] Some of the biological reasoning makes common sense: your circulation is reduced when you're sitting down, and as a result the flow of feel-good hormones to your brain is also reduced.

This is partly why the headlines in the past couple of years have declared inactivity, especially prolonged sitting, as the "new smoking." You may even have read articles suggesting that no matter how fit you are, if you sit for most of the day, you face a higher risk of numerous health challenges and premature death. So even if you exercise hard for an ambitious hour or more a day, you're still putting your health at risk if you're mostly stationary the rest of the day. And we all know how easy this can be if you spend your days driving in your car, working at a desk, and interacting with lots of screens, from computers and tablets to cell phones and televisions. Sitting too much despite exercise is akin to smoking despite exercise.

Being in a seated position is not in itself harmful. But sitting for prolonged periods over and over again entails biological effects that negatively influence things like blood fats, blood sugar balance, resting blood pressure, and many hormones, some of which help control your metabolism, appetite, and the volume of food you eat. The body essentially turns off at the metabolic activity level when it's idle for a long time. As your circulation slows down, your body uses less of your blood sugar and burns less fat, both of which increase your risk of heart disease and diabetes—two of our leading killers today. New science is showing the impact that being immobile has on certain genes. For example, one pivotal gene that's been identified is called lipid phosphate phosphatase 1, or LPP1. We think this gene helps to keep our cardiovascular system healthy by preventing dangerous blood clotting and inflammation. But it's significantly suppressed when the body is idle for a few hours, so it can't do its job to maintain cardio health. Even exercise won't impact this gene if the muscles have been inactive most of the day. In other words, LPP1 is apparently sensitive to sitting but resistant to exercise.

Makes me wonder: If all of the people who take vitamins and supplements stopped doing so and instead focused on increasing their movement throughout the day by just 10 percent, how much chronic disease and early death could we avoid? Probably a lot.

In 2010, the World Health Organization published its "Global Recommendations on Physical Activity for Health," which resembles the American guidelines that were last published in 2008.[4] Physical activity, the WHO pointed out, is the fourth leading risk factor for global mortality. And sedentary living is unfortunately on the rise across the globe. When you look at the top five risk factors for mortality, however, all of them are interrelated:

High blood pressure	13 percent
Tobacco usage	9 percent
High blood glucose	6 percent
Physical inactivity	6 percent
Overweight and obesity	5 percent

These risk factors account for nearly 40 percent of global mortality. Physical inactivity may only account for 6 percent, but it's closely related to the other factors, as it paves the way for high blood pressure, high blood glucose, and being overweight or obese. There is also evidence that exercise helps people lessen or eradicate their smoking habits. After all, when you exercise regularly, you tend to avoid activities that send your health in the other direction. With fitness comes the inspiration to eat better, move more, and generally live better.

Note that physical activity encompasses a lot of different kinds of movement. It's not just about formal exercise in a gym or going on a run. Physical activity includes, as put by the WHO, "leisure time physical activity (e.g., walking, dancing, gardening, hiking, swimming), transportation (e.g., walking or cycling), occupational (i.e., work), household chores, play, games, sports or planned exercise, in the context of daily, family, and community activities."

The science of exercise wasn't a course offered when I was in medical school. The world has changed immensely since then, and today entire new disciplines of medicine have emerged to study physiology in this regard. Metabolomics, for example, is a form of health profiling that identifies metabolic patterns in people that either heighten or lower their risk for certain illnesses. Scientists can get a chemical snapshot of the effects of exercise by examining blood samples. This kind of research has led to the discovery that the fitter you are, the more your body and its myriad systems benefit, thanks to dramatic changes that happen spontaneously during physical movement.

I marvel at the fact that we've only recently realized, from a scientific standpoint, the power of movement over time. In 2012, it was finally shown just how many years of life can be gained after age forty as a result of various levels of physical activity, both overall and according to body mass index (BMI).[5] The conclusions emerged from six studies in the National Cancer Institute Cohort Consortium, comprising 654,827 individuals from twenty-one years of age all the way up to ninety. The following graph reveals the research's findings:

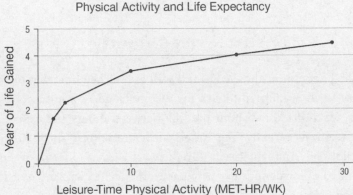

Physical Activity and Life Expectancy

Leisure-time physical activity is associated with longer life expectancy, even at relatively low levels of activity and regardless of body weight.

Metabolic equivalent hours per week (MET-h/wk) is how the researchers calculated the extent of the participants' exercise. A physical activity level of 0.1 to 3.74 MET-h/wk, for instance, is the same as brisk walking for up to 75 minutes per week. Higher levels of physical activity were associated with greater gains in life expectancy, with a gain of 4.5 years at the highest level (22.5+ MET-h/wk, equivalent to brisk walking for 450+ minutes per week, which is 7½ hours). Substantial gains were also recorded in each BMI group. In joint analyses, being active (7.5+ MET-h/wk) and normal weight (BMI 18.5–24.9) was correlated with a gain of 7.2 years of life compared to being inactive (0 MET-h/wk) and obese (BMI 35.0+). A BMI of 35+ in an inactive individual was actually shown to be associated with seven years of life lost compared to meeting recommended activity levels and being normal weight.

So it's a foregone conclusion: a physically active lifestyle is vital for good health as well as important for increasing life expectancy. What probably surprised some of the researchers is that the people who were overweight (but not obese) and engaged in physical activity lived longer than those of normal weight who were inactive. Other research has also shown this to be true: it's better to be physically fit and overweight than to be of normal weight and sedentary. Indeed, movement matters. Movement over time matters most.

Sitting Not So Pretty

While it's common knowledge and well established now that physical fitness levels are related to risk for metabolic and cardiovascular diseases, we didn't know about the link between fitness and cancer risk until relatively recently. The American Institute for Cancer Research now links physical activity with a reduced risk for most forms of cancer. Extended sitting periods in particular are associated with increased risk of both breast and colon cancers.

According to a study published in 2015, men with a high fitness level in midlife appear to be at lower risk for lung, colorectal, and prostate cancer, and that higher fitness level also may put them at lower risk of death if they are diagnosed with cancer when they are older.[6] The explanation for the relationship between exercise and lower risk for cancer is based on the fact that physical activity does things to the body that prevent cancer from starting or progressing. It helps control energy levels and weight, balance the body's hormonal system, regulate insulin, reduce inflammation, and influence the immune system positively. Moreover, because exercise gets your circulation going at a faster clip, there's less likelihood for toxic substances to accumulate and trigger adverse cellular reactions.

In another related study, also published in 2015, researchers showed how influential exercise can be when someone is undergoing chemotherapy for cancer.[7] Perhaps nothing can be more frustrating for doctors like me than trying to treat a cancer that continues to become increasingly stealthier, evading the drugs we throw at it. Cancers grow resistant to treatment in many ways, one of which is by generating a network of blood vessels that become so entangled that they suffocate the tumor, depriving it of oxygen. And an oxygen-starved tumor then gains a kind of shield that protects it from chemotherapy drugs and radiation, which are designed to seek out well-oxygenated tissue. In research circles, we've long tested various approaches to improving blood flow to tumors in the hopes of improving treatments. Nothing has worked well, until researchers led by Duke Cancer Institute (DCI) studied the effects of exercise in mice made to model breast cancer cases in humans. They found that physical activity stimulated significant improvements in the number and function of blood vessels surrounding tumors, boosting oxygen flow to the cancer site. When blasted with chemotherapy, the tumors shrank much better in these exercising animals than they did in sedentary ones. The scientists employed two different models of breast cancer cells, implanting them in mice and then making some of them run on a wheel while allowing others to remain sedentary.

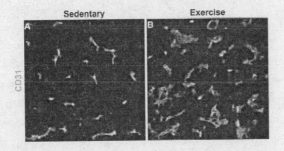

The light gray areas are the tumor blood vessels. The exercise group had significantly better blood supply in the tumor compared with the sedentary group.

Tumor growth was significantly slower among the animals that exercised than in the sedentary mice. The death of cancer cells was in fact 1.5 times higher in the exercisers. Mice that ran on the wheel developed small blood vessels that were about 60 percent higher in density compared to the sedentary controls', thereby leading to improved oxygen transport and less oxygen starvation to the tumor.

Next, the researchers looked at whether exercise would improve chemotherapy. The mice were randomly assigned to one of four groups: sedentary, exercise alone, chemo alone, or exercise in combination with the chemotherapy. The rate of cancer growth was dramatically delayed in mice treated with exercise and chemo compared to all of the other groups. Cancer growth was also slowed in both the exercise alone and chemo alone groups, but there was no difference in tumor growth rate between those two groups. This observation suggested that exercise has a similar effect to chemotherapy. What exercise was doing, essentially, was changing the body's context—changing the environment in a way that made it less hospitable for the tumor to grow.

Earlier studies have confirmed that people who are fitter during their thirties through their fifties have less chronic illness in later years. One of these studies in particular, published in the *Archives of Internal Medicine* in 2012, looked at 18,670 participants in the Cooper Center Longitudinal Study, which contained records of more than 250,000 patients over forty years.[8] They compared the data with the participants' Medicare claims during the ages of seventy to eighty-five. The results were similar in both men and women:

People who increased their fitness levels by 20 percent in their midlife years decreased their chances of developing chronic illness by 20 percent in old age. When the individuals turned fifty, the part of the group in the bottom 20 percent of the fitness scale had almost *twice* as many chronic illnesses as those in the top 20 percent. People with the highest fitness levels at midlife enjoyed more time being illness-free than those who were the least fit. Fitter people also lived their last five years with fewer chronic diseases.

Just how much time do we spend in a parked position? According to one team of researchers at Louisiana's Pennington Biomedical Research Center who published their findings in 2012, whether or not people exercise the recommended 150 minutes a week, we spend an average of 64 hours a week sitting, 28 hours standing, and 11 hours moving and walking in ways that don't count as exercise.[9] That means that no matter how active we are otherwise, most of us are sitting for more than nine hours a day. Although this group's calculations were based on women, it likely reflects what's happening with men as well. One observation made by these researchers that they didn't expect is that the individuals who exercised the most didn't spend less time sitting. Regular exercisers were actually prone to making less of an effort to move outside their designated workout time. Other research has shown that people are about 30 percent less active overall on days when they do set aside time for a formal workout, as opposed to the days when they don't plan an exercise routine.

What all this translates to is a concern not only for those who don't exercise at all, but also for people who lack general movement on a regular basis to counteract all the harm that can result from sitting for most of the day. Multiple effects happen simultaneously when the body is on the go, even if it's just walking around while talking on the phone, taking the stairs instead of the elevator, or simply making a point to get up every hour for a five-minute stroll, stretch, or jog in place. All of these movements will have positive biological effects to offset the poison of excessive sitting. It doesn't help that our social infrastructure accommodates idleness. We have LEED (Leadership in Energy and Environmental Design) standards for the environmental impact of buildings, so why don't we establish "LHD" (Leadership in Health Design) standards for office buildings also? This can entail any number of innovations, such as more openly accessible staircases, in-house gyms, and nutritious food served in cafés and commissaries. We have become a society in which the more important you are, the closer your parking space is to your desk, and the more resources you have, the more bathrooms your family enjoys so no one has to walk far to use one. We need to change this thinking and develop building codes and incentives that reflect a new understanding of health.

Don't let appearances skew your perception of fitness. There are a lot of people today who embody the so-called lean paradox, which refers to the way thin people can look healthy on the outside but be suffering from many health problems on the inside. These individuals may try to manage their weight and health through diet alone, shunning physical activity. They lose out on exercise's metabolic benefits, and they experience consequences similar to those they would if they were morbidly obese.

Strength training becomes more important the older we get, as we naturally lose muscle mass and strength. Strength typically peaks between thirty-five and forty years of age. After that, we start losing about 1 percent of our strength per year. That rate picks up speed in our seventies and eighties. Strength training supports muscle mass, can help rebuild it, and can help increase bone mass. The muscles we employ when we lift a weight put pressure on our bones, forcing them to get stronger. Muscle mass and strength are among the most underappreciated and unrecognized aspects of health.

Why Loss of Muscle Can Lead to Loss of Life

Muscle plays key roles in the body beyond the obvious ones like helping us stand erect and move; just as fat stores extra calories for energy reserves, muscle serves as an emergency supply of the amino acids we need to build tissues and biological substances. The body doesn't store amino acids as it does fat and carbs; if there's not enough coming in from the diet, the body will take them from its own tissue by breaking down its protein sources, usually muscle. Which is partly why loss of muscle can lead to loss of life.

In 2006, Robert Wolfe, who is now director of the Center for Translational Research in Aging and Longevity at the University of Arkansas for Medical Sciences, wrote a paper for *The American Journal of Clinical Nutrition* titled "The Underappreciated Role of Muscle in Health and Disease," in which he chronicled muscle's role in the body.[10] Over the past several decades Dr. Wolfe has performed pioneering research in human metabolism, especially as it relates to aging and specific medical problems. In this particular publication, in which muscle is described as the unsung hero, he emphasizes muscle's contribution to the prevention of many common conditions and chronic diseases. His paper echoes what other scientists have found when they examine the biological benefits of muscle and muscular strength.

More muscular strength has been shown to be associated with the following:

- smaller waist circumference
- less weight and fat gain
- lower risk of developing hypertension
- less insulin resistance
- lower chronic inflammation
- lower risk of high blood pressure
- lower levels of triglyceride (blood fats)
- lower levels of bad (LDL) cholesterol
- better blood sugar balance

Contrary to what you might think, recovering from illness or trauma relies a lot on muscle mass, muscle strength, and muscle function. Multiple studies have demonstrated that muscle mass and strength factor into how long it takes to recuperate from illness or injury. The less muscle mass and strength before, the longer to return to a normal life, if that's even possible. I see this frequently among cancer patients. The ones diagnosed with cancer who are physically strong live longer than those who enter a period of illness frail.

While it's common knowledge now that chronic diseases related to poor lifestyle account for many deaths in the United States, it's not widely understood that changes in muscle play an important role in the progression of most conditions. Take, for example, the damaging effects of advanced heart disease and cancer. Both of these illnesses are often associated with rapid loss of muscle mass and metabolic function, and survival can often depend on the extent of muscle loss.

Because aging involves a gradual muscle loss over time that speeds up as one gets older, there's a relationship between the state of one's muscle mass and length of life. The progressive loss of muscle mass and function that typically occurs with aging is called sarcopenia, and it can erode one's quality of life over time. Imagine not being able to do basic activities like getting out of bed, walking, feeding yourself, or using and moving your body to take care of yourself. A devastating loss of muscle mass can lead to such an outcome. Muscle mass and strength are key to survival, arguably as fundamental as oxygen and water, food and sleep. And losing them isn't inevitable!

A 2011 study out of the University of Pittsburgh subjected a cross-section of 40 high-level recreational athletes, who were aged forty to eighty-one years and trained four to five times per week, to a battery of tests to demonstrate that muscle strength does not have to decline significantly with age.[11] Their results contradicted the common belief that muscle mass and strength decline automatically as a function of aging. The researchers noted that such declines may signal the effect of chronic *disuse* rather than muscle aging. They wrote: "This maintenance of muscle mass and strength may decrease or eliminate the falls, functional decline, and loss of independence that are commonly seen in aging adults."

Movement All Day Keeps the Doctor Away

A question that science has been trying to answer is what the perfect dose of exercise should be. So many things in health and medicine come with dosing instructions, but not exercise. And even though we're told to spend at least 150 minutes engaged in moderate exercise per week, that guideline is so broad as to be meaningless to most people. Exercise has had a "Goldilocks problem," with experts wrestling with finding the line between too much and too little.[12]

Although the sweet spot for any individual will be different, the data from two recent large-scale studies suggests that, generally speaking, the ideal amount of exercise for a long life is a little more than what many of us think, but we don't have to run marathons. And if we do like to take exercise to extremes, the latest research also shows that intense or prolonged exercise is not likely to be harmful and could extend people's lives by years.

These impressive studies were published in 2015 in *JAMA Internal Medicine*. One of them, conducted by researchers with the National Cancer Institute, Harvard University, and other institutions, collected information about people's exercise habits from six large, ongoing health surveys.[13] They managed to gather data from more than 661,000 adults. Then, the researchers created categories for these people based on how much they exercised on a weekly basis. There were those who didn't work out at all and some who exercised to extremes—working out for twenty-five hours per week or more, ten times the current recommendations. Comparing fourteen years' worth of death records for these different groups, all of which were made up mostly of middle-aged folks, the researchers found that the people who didn't exercise at all were at the highest risk of premature death. Not so surprising. But what was interesting is that those who did some form of exercise below the recommendations lowered their risk of an early death by 20 percent. That's a huge benefit for a little bit of effort. The individuals who completed the recommended 150 minutes per week of moderate exercise of course showed greater longevity benefits. These folks enjoyed 31 percent less risk of dying during the fourteen-year period compared with the people who never exercised.

The optimal amount of time, however, to gain the most benefits was found to be 450 minutes per week, which is a little more than an hour a day. According to the data, the people who tripled the recommended level of exercise were 39 percent less likely to meet an early death than people who never exercised. And they weren't spending this time running at full speed or maxing out their heart rate on a piece of gym equipment. They were working out moderately, mostly by walking. This was where the benefits hit their peak, though they didn't necessarily take a total U-turn thereafter. The few people who took their exercise time to extremes, at least ten times the 150-minute recommendation, enjoyed roughly the same reduction in mortality risk as those who simply met the guidelines, but not as much as the 450-minute group. In other words, they didn't increase their risk of a premature death, but they didn't bank more health benefits for all those extra minutes breaking more sweat.

The second study, from Australia, shared a similar conclusion, though it was more focused on determining how intensity factors into the mortality equation.[14] And it debunked the conventional wisdom that says frequent, strenuous exercise might contribute to an early death. Much to the contrary, the study found that spending lots of time engaged in a strenuous activity increases longevity. As with the other study, the researchers first categorized the people in their sample, a batch of more than 200,000 middle-aged Australian adults followed for more than six years, based on how much time they spent exercising and at what intensity level. They wanted to see the difference between people who engaged in only moderate activity (e.g., social tennis, gentle swimming, or light household chores) and those who included at least some vigorous activity (e.g., competitive tennis, aerobics, jogging). Checking death statistics, the researchers confirmed what the other study concluded: meeting the exercise guidelines lowered the risk of premature death by a lot. This held true even for people whose exercise was simply walking.

What probably surprised the researchers is that adding intensity—but not necessarily more time sweating—conferred substantial benefits. The people who spent up to 30 percent of their weekly workouts in strenuous activities were 9 percent less likely to die sooner than expected as compared to those who exercised *for the same amount of time* with no vigorous activity. And those who engaged in strenuous activities for more than 30 percent of their exercise time earned an extra 13 percent reduction in early death, compared with the group who had no vigorous activity. For the small handful of folks who spent more than 30 percent of their workout doing intense exercise, no corresponding increase in mortality was noted.

The only big caveat to these studies' conclusions is that the researchers had to rely on people's memories about their exercise habits. In other words, these were observational studies and not randomized experiments. So they can't definitely prove a causal relationship between any exercise dose and changes in mortality risk, but there was enough evidence to say that exercise and death risks are associated. And the associations are indeed strong and consistent enough to say that movement, and vigorous movement once in a while, does a body good.

Even though I asked you to track your movement during the two-week challenge, you might still be wondering how fit you are today. And you might also question whether you're in the bottom 20 percent.

In general, if you can walk a couple of miles at a decent pace, cover-
ing a mile per fifteen minutes, or climb several flights of stairs without
difficulty, then you are in average shape at any age, whether you're a
man or woman. But there's usually room for improvement. In terms of
muscle mass, you've probably got some decent muscle strength if you
can complete your normal daily activities without much strain. But
again, there's always room for improvement.

I'll also give you a quick fitness test to do right now: Using the least
amount of support that you need and without worrying about how fast
you're moving, can you sit on the floor and then rise up to a standing
position? Turns out that if you can get yourself up from the floor using
just one hand—or even better, without the help of any hand—then you
are not only in the top 25 percent of musculoskeletal fitness, but your
survival prognosis is probably better than that of those unable to do
so. In 2012, a study performed in Brazil at an exercise medicine clinic
revealed that an inability to sit and rise from the floor shows an all-cause
mortality risk (another way of saying that you're more likely to die from
any cause).[15] Put simply, the better you can do this task without relying
on your hands for stability and support, the longer you'll live.

You don't need to sign up for an athletic event or join a running
group to attain an ideal level of fitness. In the empowering words of leg-
endary University of Oregon track and field coach and Nike cofounder
Bill Bowerman, "If you have a body, you are an athlete." Although we
all would do well to maintain a formal exercise program that builds
and maintains fitness through a combination of cardio work, strength
training, and stretching, a more fundamental and primary goal should
be just moving more throughout the day. You should make it a goal to
become at least 10 percent fitter than you are today.

You can engage in short bursts of exercise throughout the day, which
can help minimize your time spent sitting. Or you can commit to a routine that blocks out an hour or so for your workouts. Just be sure that if
you do dedicate a single period to your exercise regimen, you don't allow
yourself to be sedentary the rest of the day. Ideally, break up your sitting
time by getting up and walking periodically (remember, how fast you

can walk is a signal of future health). Keep a pair of three- or five-pound free weights near your desk to perform some bicep curls on a break.

In the Lucky Years, technology will increasingly help us be less sedentary and stay fitter, and keep track of these metrics. If you completed the two-week challenge I outlined in chapter 5, you know you can monitor how much you move during the day and record levels of exertion. Whether you use the most complicated or the simplest technologies, monitoring your body's movement over time is key to understanding it. Health and fitness apps can tell you more than you ever wanted to know about yourself, giving you truly objective data that can help you plan your workouts and maximize opportunities to move. Be careful not to overwhelm yourself with too many apps and gadgetry, however. You risk burning out on all that tracking and quickly losing interest as fast as you can with a fad diet. Start with basic apps that will track your mileage and minutes in a state of heightened heartbeats. Then add more apps and gadgets as you go along and find technologies that you know you will use. One site to bookmark is Greatist.com. It offers a catalog of the best health and fitness apps and will help you navigate all the latest and greatest tools. It covers all kinds of health-related apps, including those in the categories of food and nutrition, mind and brain, sleep, and productivity.

Antiaging Hoaxes

Before I end this chapter, I must throw in a little bit about popular strategies to look and feel younger. These include things like testosterone and human growth hormone pills and injections. You know I'm not going to endorse the use of the products that come with significant risk factors. Case in point: Contrary to what the multibillion-dollar testosterone-boosting drug industry claims, these drugs have not been shown to reverse common issues related to aging such as low libido, fatigue, and muscle loss. Yet they come with potentially serious long-term complications, chiefly cardiovascular problems.

Testosterone therapy was developed for people who had pituitary problems—people who made no testosterone at all. Over the last decade, though, people started to use it for all the problems of aging, even though medical science does not support that. In fall 2014, the FDA moved to change the labeling on the drug, thereby drastically limiting its use to men who have abnormally low hormone levels due to disease or injury, instead of aging. This $2 billion industry was examined in a 2015 *Journal of the American Medical Association* study on patients with low-testosterone (or Low-T). It found that the testosterone gel administration did not improve overall sexual function or health-related quality of life, the reason most of the men were taking the supplementation.

Clearly, the body ages. It's a normal physiological process. Hormone levels change, cells don't turn over as fast, and we don't bounce back as easily the older we get. It's normal and natural to age. I have faith that one day we'll be able to change the effects and tempo of aging through some of the therapies I've already described, such as turning on sleeping stem cells and leveraging the body's internal machinery naturally. But to try to reverse aging through synthetic antiaging drugs is cheating the system. There are ramifications. After all, there's a reason the body doesn't produce the same amount of growth hormone when you're seventy as when you were seven. That growth hormone is spurring development in the youngster; in the older adult, it's also stimulating growth but at a huge physiological cost. And if that older adult happens to have any cancerous cells growing, guess what that supplemental growth hormone is doing: Acting like Miracle-Gro.

Any kind of hormone therapy used to combat the effects of aging should be suspect. We all want to look and feel younger, but there are better ways to achieve that goal without compromising your system's natural process. The real antiaging secret is using proven metrics to optimize your health, like eating dinner before seven in the evening to get a good night's sleep or taking a 20-minute walk at two in the afternoon to beat the midday lull and resist the craving for a sugar fix. With technologies to help us stay attuned to ourselves, we can effect positive changes to our body's system without artificially tinkering with it. And as you're about to find out, whatever we can do to tame inflammation will go a long way to keeping us looking and feeling as young as can be.

CHAPTER 8

Wonder Drugs That Work

Sleep, Sex, Touching, and Tools to Tame Inflammation

Our bodies are our gardens, to the which our wills are gardeners.

—William Shakespeare, *Othello*, act I, scene III

The next time you're at a high-stakes baseball game or watching one on TV, think about all that went into preparing for the game, from equipment to strategy, coaching and consulting. I bet that among the things that cross your mind, seeking advice from sleep experts is not on the list.

In April of 2015, Matt McCarthy, a doctor himself, reported on an unusual story for *Sports Illustrated*: Major League Baseball's experiments with sleep.[1] Put another way, his article covered the league's attempt to manage "circadian disadvantages"—sleep deprivation due to traveling across time zones and the impact on a player's performance.

At the heart of McCarthy's reporting was the story of Red Sox's first baseman Mike Napoli, who underwent surgery in 2013 to reconfigure his chin, jaw, and sinuses to help him breathe easier at night. Napoli had suffered from a very common sleep disorder called sleep apnea since his early twenties. The disorder causes the airway to collapse during sleep when the muscles in the back of the throat fail to keep the airway open. So your breathing essentially gets cut off multiple times, your sleep becomes fragmented, and your blood is not as oxygenated as it should be. Loud snoring and dreamless sleep are often telltale signs of sleep apnea. Napoli couldn't recall a dream in more than a decade before his surgery fixed his problem. Sufferers of sleep apnea who don't receive treatment never feel fully rested, and this can result in chronic sleep deprivation that raises risks for a slew of health conditions, from hypertension and heart disease to mood and memory problems.

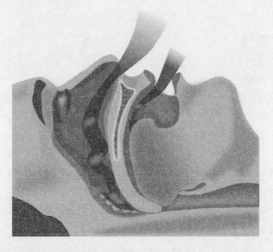

An illustration of how sleep apnea happens and how the air breathed in can be blocked by the position of the throat. Sleep apnea is caused by the muscles of the upper respiratory system relaxing. The throat then becomes narrow or even completely blocked, which doesn't allow enough air to pass, leading to loud snoring noises when the individual breathes in and out. As a result, the body does not get enough oxygen.

In 2015, an alarming new study published in *Neurology* found that sleep apnea doesn't just casually hasten memory and thinking declines as if you're having a benign "senior moment."[2] It may in fact lead to earlier diagnoses of mild cognitive impairment (MCI) and Alzheimer's disease; MCI is often a precursor to dementia. The New York University researchers of this particular study found that patients with sleep apnea were, on average, diagnosed with mild cognitive impairment nearly ten years earlier than those who didn't suffer from breathing problems during their sleep. The time span for developing Alzheimer's also seemed to speed up: those with sleep apnea were diagnosed, on average, five years sooner than were sound sleepers. Among the theories given to explain this connection are the adverse effects of oxygen loss on the brain, as well as the fact that sleep entails a slew of physiological events that help the brain to "freshen up," do some housecleaning, and clear out proteins that can otherwise gunk up nerve cells.

For professional athletes in their prime, major sleep deprivation can be destructive to performance. Although it hasn't been shown to impact muscle strength, it can impair reflexes, judgment, healing, attention, and motivation, all of which are key ingredients to success on a court, field, or racecourse. By some measures, chronic sleep deprivation can slow reaction times nearly tenfold, so imagine that kind of impact on a Major League Baseball player who has just fractions of a second to decide whether to swing at a fast curveball. Dr. Scott Kutscher, a neurologist and sleep expert at Vanderbilt University Medical Center, has looked at players' behavior while up to bat, measuring a player's tendency to swing at pitches outside of the strike zone (what's also called plate discipline). Kutscher argues that for many players, their discipline in this regard becomes progressively worse over the course of a season. And he's convinced that this has to do with fatigue, which impairs judgment.

Dr. Christopher Winter, board certified in both neurology and sleep medicine, is medical director of Charlottesville Neurology and Sleep Medicine in Virginia. His landmark 2009 study put time zones and baseball players to the test when he looked at how traveling across time zones for games impacted players and the outcomes of their performances.[3] After evaluating ten seasons (that's over the course of ten years), he found that if a team crossed a time zone to play a game, it was at a slight disadvantage compared to a visiting team that did not deal with a time change. And a team that crossed three time zones had a less than 50 percent chance of victory. The reason for this weakness is a disruption in circadian rhythm—the body's internal clock that revolves around its sleep/wake cycles and is paced by environmental cues such as light and temperature, as well as the hormone melatonin. Dr. Winter's work has inspired a number of Major League teams to find the secret sauce to fight fatigue and leverage the circadian *advantage*—being in the right place at the right time to perform optimally. Interestingly, his research has also revealed that players who wrestle with sleep depriva- tion don't typically stay in Major League Baseball as long as those who get their beauty (er, athletic) sleep. When the Giants consulted with Winter during the World Series in 2014, the team opted to spend the night in Missouri after a game rather than fly home that night. The fol- lowing week they won the Series.

The idea that a well-rested ballplayer is more likely to be a win- ning ballplayer is the example we need to keep in mind for all of us, no matter what we do for a living or what kind of performances we're giving in our personal and professional lives. According to the National Institutes of Health, chronic problems with sleep that can significantly diminish health, alertness, and safety affect up to 70 million Americans. The number of chronic diseases linked to chronic sleep deprivation and untreated sleep disorders is astounding. In addition to the ones I've already mentioned, others include uncontrollable weight manage- ment, stroke, diabetes, and cancer. If colds haunt you throughout the year, perhaps it's because you're not getting enough shut-eye; in 2015 a group of researchers confirmed that people who are "short-sleepers," meaning they sleep six hours a night or less, are more than four times more likely to catch a cold, compared to those who get more than seven hours in a night. In fact, Centers for Disease Control and Prevention considers insufficient sleep a public-health epidemic. From a scientific perspective, sleep is emerging as so potent a factor in better health that we need to view it as a nonnegotiable priority and install policies to support it. It may be among the lowest-tech strategies we have at our disposal to enhance the quality of our life and health in the Lucky Years.

And there won't ever be a gizmo, gadget, or drug we can take to negate our need for sleep or replicate its benefits on the body.

Most people know when to seek medical help for pain or unexplained symptoms that disrupt their daily life. But sleep problems are often ignored or overlooked. Which is why the overwhelming majority of people with sleep disorders do not seek treatment and are not diagnosed.

In 2015, the National Sleep Foundation (NSF), along with a group of experts, issued its new recommendations for sleep. The report suggests wider sleep ranges for most age groups. The NSF arrived at these updated figures after they formed a panel from various fields including pediatrics, neurology, gerontology, and gynecology to reach a consensus. The panel revised the recommended sleep ranges for all six children and teenage groups. A summary of the new recommendations includes: [4]

Newborns (0 to 3 months): Sleep range narrowed to
   14 to 17 hours each day (previously it was 12 to 18).
Infants (4 to 11 months): Sleep range widened two hours to
   12 to 15 hours (previously it was 14 to 15).
Toddlers (1 to 2 years): Sleep range widened by one hour to
   11 to 14 hours (previously it was 12 to 14).
Preschoolers (3 to 5): Sleep range widened by one hour to
   10 to 13 hours (previously it was 11 to 13).
School-age children (6 to 13): Sleep range widened by one hour
   to 9 to 11 hours (previously it was 10 to 11).
Teenagers (14 to 17): Sleep range widened by one hour to
   8 to 10 hours (previously it was 8.5 to 9.5).
Younger adults (18 to 25): Sleep range is 7 to 9 hours
   (new age category).
Adults (26 to 64): Sleep range did not change and remains
   7 to 9 hours.
Older adults (65+): Sleep range is 7 to 8 hours
   (new age category).

I'll admit that I may preach the value of restful sleep but find myself equally challenged by the task of achieving high-quality sleep on a routine basis. I'm constantly at the mercy of an unforgiving work schedule and commitments to events that often require me to make long trips across multiple time zones or get up super early after an evening dinner I had to attend. But I do my best, and I know that I don't suffer from any serious sleep disorder. That's the first thing you can do if you find yourself routinely sleep deprived: focus on your nightly slumber and find out if you have a problem that should be addressed by a physician. Does it take more than twenty or thirty minutes to fall asleep? Do you wake up in the middle of the night and have a hard time falling back asleep? Has anyone told you that you snore?

We live in a world that makes sleep look outdated, undesirable, and optional. With our overscheduled lives, 24-7 access to media, screens, online retail, and artificial light, and our urge to check our phones and emails constantly, it's no wonder we suffer from a lack of sleep.

But I can't tell you how many times I've cured someone's low energy and chronic exhaustion by suggesting they get their sleep habits under control and maintain a regular schedule. One of the most commanding roles sleep has is its ability to dictate our hormonal balance—from hormones that control appetite to hormones that help us manage stress, replenish cells, heal and fight infections, utilize energy efficiently, control weight, renew skin and bones, lower risk factors for heart disease and stroke, sharpen our planning and memory skills, improve concentration, and return organ and tissue function to more youthful states.

So while you may think that your body is powered down for the night when the lights go out, that couldn't be further from the truth when it comes to what your brain is doing. It's catching its breath. It's the command center where a legion of neurons spring into action as soon as you surrender to sleep. This is when metaphorical data processors in your brain go through all the information that your brain took in that day and organize it so you can take in more and learn more the following day. This is also when your brain runs through its trusty checklist to ensure your hormones, enzymes, and proteins are balanced and in sync. Meanwhile, the brain's janitors are at work to sweep out any toxic debris that can gum up its systems if left to build up.

Sigrid Veasey is a leading sleep researcher and a professor of medicine at Perelman School of Medicine at the University of Pennsylvania. She's been working with mice to understand just what happens when the brain doesn't get its break to conduct certain business. Using her mouse models, she's found that when the brain is kept alert by neurons firing constantly, these brain cells shed free radicals as a byproduct of making energy.[5] Free radicals are rogue molecules that have lost an electron and thus they are highly reactive in the body, damaging healthy cells and tissues. They can potentially be toxic to the brain if they are not swept up. And it turns out that during sleep, these same neurons also produce antioxidants that take care of these free radicals. But periods of sleep loss, even if they are brief, can be damaging: the cells fail to make enough antioxidants to counter the buildup of free radicals. As a result, some of the neurons die and they cannot be recovered. After several weeks of depriving her mice of adequate sleep, the mice "are more likely to be sleepy when they are supposed to be active and have more difficulty consolidating [the benefits of] sleep during their sleep period."[6]

Veasey thinks that the same sequence of events happens in aging brains. As neurons become less adept at cleaning up their waste, they poison themselves. So a good question is: What are we doing to our brains when we don't get enough sleep? If we suffer from chronic sleep deprivation, are we simultaneously aging our brains prematurely? Is it possible for the brain of a thirty-year-old to look more like that of a sixty-year-old? Some of the research is already showing that yes, this might be true. After all, if sleep didn't have value, then it would be one of evolution's biggest and most inefficient mistakes!

In research performed by Maiken Nedergaard, codirector of the Center for Translational Neuromedicine at the University of Rochester, it's been found that nonneuronal glial cells in the brain, which hadn't been given much attention previously in research circles, act as little pumps when the body sleeps.[7] All organs use energy, but perhaps none so much as the brain. And in the process of using energy, organs create waste products. Most organs sweep away their own garbage with the help of an efficient system nearby, such as by recruiting specialized immune cells that can chew up the trash like a disposal. Some organs are tied into a mesh of vessels that are part of the lymph system, the body's drainage pipes.

Although we just recently discovered in 2015 that the brain is connected directly to the immune system by lymphatic vessels we didn't know existed before, the brain isn't couched in lymph vessels like other parts of the body.[8] During our wakeful hours, it's the glial cells that help the brain's neurons carry out their main function: firing electrical impulses and transmitting signals. Because glial cells can't conduct neuronal activity, they were ignored for a long time by neuroscientists. But then Nedergaard, a busy mother who wanted to get to the bottom of why the brain needs sleep, discovered that glial cells aren't as static and boring as previously thought. With the help of clinical trials on mice, she noticed that as soon as a mouse fell asleep, the glial cells would take center stage, turning the volume way down on the brain's electrical activity.

There's a dramatic and measurable difference between a brain that's operating in a person fully awake versus someone in deep slumber. The wakeful brain "resembles a busy airport, swelling with the cumulative activity of individual messages traveling from one neuron to another. The activity inflates the size of brain cells until they take up 86 percent of the brain's volume."[9] The sleeping brain, on the other hand, is characterized by repetitive cycles of low firing and nonexistent firing of neurons depending on which stage of sleep the brain is in. Meanwhile, the brain's cells shrink in size to make room for the fluid in between them to cleanse the system.

"It's like a dishwasher that keeps flushing through to wash the dirt away," says Nedergaard.[10] This purifying action also goes on when we're awake, but not at the same level of intensity. All of which is to say that when we don't get enough sleep, we don't experience that high level of detoxification in the brain thanks to those glial cells. Such findings have gotten neuroscientists curious as to whether sleep deprivation contributes to degenerative brain disorders, especially if they occur earlier in life than expected.

Both Nedergaard's and Veasey's work also points to why older brains are more susceptible to developing dementia such as Alzheimer's disease, which may be caused by hostile proteins that aren't cleared quickly enough. The molecular trash builds up, but the garbage collectors are not picking up fast enough, so the trash continues to pile up and adversely affect nearby cells and their functionality.

Most people don't like to be told that sleep is often the quickest and easiest way to regulate their bodies and feel a positive difference in a short time. They'd rather take a shortcut through pills, caffeine, or sugar than be told to sleep better. Even in the Lucky Years, with lots of revolutionary technologies and medicines available, we need to respect and practice good sleep hygiene. While plenty of things can knock us out, nothing can replicate all of sleep's benefits. We've spent decades trying to find a way to package the benefits of sleep into a pill, but it hasn't happened and probably never will. It's fine to track and monitor your sleep using apps and technologies, but aim to achieve restful, all-natural sleep as much as possible. Although there will always be some genetic mutant who can get by on just a few hours of sleep a night, just as there will always be someone who can run faster than you, the vast majority of us need at least seven hours of shut-eye.

Remember, sleep is just one activity in the chain of events you undergo each day that contributes or takes away from your health. What you do during the day will undoubtedly affect your sleep at night. As I've said throughout, regularity 24-7 is the goal. Far too often, we learn to suppress our body's preferred schedule to meet goals that might satisfy other areas of our lives but shift us further from health.

Sexual Healing

Speaking of sleep, I should mention the other activity related to the bedroom that confers substantial health benefits: sex. Beyond just helping us sleep, sex is an activity whose frequency and satisfaction can be considered a vital sign of health, but its benefits can be downplayed in our society as much as sleep.

I'll preface this section with what should be the obvious: I'm referring to healthy sexual habits that eliminate risk for the transfer of disease. And I'm talking about consensual sex between two people.

Although sex is touted to relieve stress, reduce pain, ease depression, strengthen blood vessels, boost the immune system, and lower the risk of prostate and breast cancer (not to mention improve sleep and burn calories), a good question is: Does sex actually make people healthier or do healthier people have more sex?

It turns out that not only is that a difficult question to answer scientifically, but all the claims about the benefits of sex are not that easy to prove on a purely scientific basis, meaning one backed by randomized, double-blind, placebo-controlled studies. More research is needed. Dr. Irwin Goldstein, a urologist and editor in chief of the *Journal of Sexual Medicine*, stated it best when he said: "The biggest obstacle is lack of funding. If 'sex' is in your grant proposal, it's very hard to get it approved."[11] Goldstein is also president and director of the Institute for Sexual Medicine in San Diego.

I don't think we need scientific proof to show what most of us have experienced when it comes to sex. Under the right circumstances (i.e., good sex), it feels good and life seems great. We experience both a relaxation and satiation response. Now, scientifically speaking, there are biochemicals involved. Sexual activity entails a chemical cascade of hormones and neurotransmitters that can have lasting effects. Arousal increases dopamine, which activates the brain's reward centers—the same places that create positive feelings upon eating dessert or winning a hand in Vegas. After orgasm, dopamine levels drop and prolactin levels rise to bring on feelings of satisfaction and sleepiness, particularly in men. Sex also increases oxytocin, the bonding hormone that reduces fear and stimulates endorphins, our body's natural painkillers.

As with so many things in life and health, the "more is better" recommendation doesn't even apply to something as pleasurable and innocuous as sex. Decades of research show that the satisfaction and meaning you attach to sex are what's important. Put simply, if you're enjoying your sex life and it's compatible with who you are, then it doesn't get much better than that, and you don't need to change anything. Ramping up your sexual activity isn't going to make you any healthier. And even though there will be an endless number of studies that say people who have sex four or five times a week are happier and earn more money, these things are affected by many other factors. Nonetheless, sexual activity is an important player in our personal health and, from a broader perspective, our social welfare. It influences us throughout our life span. It's also the behavior that affords us the ability to experience the granddaddy of the senses: touch.

Touchy Feely

The power of touch is a sorely underappreciated aspect of intimacy that confers substantial health benefits and doesn't have to be sexual. Our need for touch is so compelling a hunger, in fact, that both animals and humans die for lack of it. Perhaps that is why the body has developed a special reflex to preserve the sense of touch when faced with something that might damage it, such as a hot stove. Your hand pulls away quicker than you can consciously think about the fact that the stove is dangerously hot.

Clearly, when you're in an intimate setting with a loved one, whether it's sexual in nature or not, skin-to-skin contact is often part of the experience. Only in the past couple of decades have we come to understand the true power of touch, starting with the landmark studies done in the mid-1990s by Harvard's Mary Carlson, a neurobiologist who measured stress in Romanian children raised in orphanages or attending poor-quality day-care centers. Carlson performed her work during the height of the *leagăne*, which literally means "cradles" and refers to the state-run institutional homes for very young children that proliferated during this time.[12]

In the mid-1960s, Romanian Communist president Nicolae Ceauşescu had enacted ironfisted policies that forced families to bear more children than they could afford. In his attempt to increase the population to boost industrial output, not only did he restrict contraceptives and ban abortions unless a woman had at least four children, but he taxed childless men and women who were over the age of twenty-five. The tax hike was a ghastly 30 percent. The birthrate rose, but not enough for him. By 1985, he took measures even further, raising the minimum number of children per couple to five and forcing women as old as forty-five to bear children.

The eventual result of Ceaușescu's brutish governance was that thousands of young children, from newborns to toddlers, were orphaned by their biological parents who could not afford to take care of them. So they were left to grow up neglected in the *leagăne,* understaffed institutions where they were deprived of adequate sensory experiences, especially that of touch. Most of the babies were abandoned right after birth in hospitals or maternity wards. After they turned three in the *leagăne,* they were transferred to another type of children's home. Much of the rest of the world didn't know this was going on until Ceaușescu was overthrown and subsequently killed in December of 1989 and images of these children finally landed on television. In 1994, Mary Carlson and her husband, Felton Earls, a Harvard psychiatrist, traveled to Romania to learn more about these children and the effects of maternal deprivation. Carlson had studied under Harry Harlow, the famous psychologist who first wrote about the impact of social deprivation following his experiments in the 1950s with monkeys. After conducting a series of observations and measurements of stress levels among Romanian children, including children in an early-enrichment program and a group of controls, Carlson concluded that the lack of touching and attention stunted the growth of the *leagăne* children and adversely affected their behavior. They'd be found rocking, swaying, staring blankly into space, and they would be disturbingly quiet and antisocial. Carlson published her results in 1997, and since then others have confirmed the overwhelming power of physical touch and attention.[13] Newer research has gone so far as to show the intricate play between our skin, the brain and nervous system, and our immunology and ability to evade or fight disease.

One of the first senses we develop is touch. It's arguably the most essential and fundamental sense for survival, stimulating our bodies in important ways throughout our lives. Different types of touch hold different meanings. Like a magic wand, touch has the power to change our heart rate, lower blood pressure and cortisol levels, spark the release of feel-good hormones and neurotransmitters, and stimulate the area of the brain that controls memory, the hippocampus.

Tiffany Field, the head of the Touch Research Institute at the University of Miami's Miller School of Medicine, has studied the sense of touch for more than thirty years. In a 2010 paper, she showed how the brain is adept at telling the difference between an emotional touch and a nonemotional one.[14] Certain touch receptors are charged with conveying emotions to the brain, while others are tasked with reporting sensory information about the external environment. It's also recently been shown that we can interpret other people's emotions based on how they touch us. And this is possible in the absence of sight—we can detect a person's basic emotions through touch without even seeing them. Emotions aren't just "touchy-feely" experiences. They are unique drivers of our behavior, shaping how we act and what we do.

In our everyday interactions, we always experience touch in context. But it's not always easy to separate touch's physical and emotional effects. In 2014, a coterie of researchers from Carnegie Mellon, the University of Virginia, and the University of Pittsburgh published results that reveal the power of hugs on the immune system.[15] Indeed, hugs may be as vital to our health as food, sleep, and water. In their experiment, they monitored 404 adults over two weeks, asking them about their daily hug counts and social interactions. Then the people were sent to rooms on an isolated hotel floor where they were exposed to a common cold virus. Most of them (78 percent) became infected, and a little more than 31 percent had the obvious signs of illness. But there was a difference between those who came down with the bug in a bad way and those who weathered the illness like it was no big deal. Those who had the most loving social interactions sailed through the infection with fewer symptoms. The researchers determined that the effects of their social support and, in particular, hugging and touching, accounted for 32 percent of the reduction effect.

In his recent book *Touch: The Science of Hand, Heart, and Mind,* the Johns Hopkins University neuroscientist David Linden summarizes the power of touch perfectly when he writes: "From consumer choice to sexual intercourse, from tool use to chronic pain to the process of healing, the genes, cells, and neural circuits involved in the sense of touch have been crucial to creating our unique human experience."[16] The more we learn about touch, the more we must acknowledge that it's a primary color in our life from womb to death, bringing healthy hues to us from a developmental, behavioral, cognitive, and emotional perspective. And I have no doubt that future technologies and therapies will leverage this great sense to treat a variety of ailments, from those that cause a great deal of pain to the nuisances of an itch and the ravages of our next topic: inflammation.

Taming Inflammation

When a retired football player gets diagnosed with Alzheimer's disease, he can point the finger at one likely suspect: inflammation. The same is true of the person with major depression, heart disease, and raging arthritis. We've known for some time now that the cornerstone of most chronic conditions, from diabetes and obesity to cancer and dementia, is inflammation—a topic I've addressed already. Controlling chronic inflammation can go a long way toward helping one to stave off illness and disease and to preserve metabolic health in the Lucky Years. So how do you do that? I have two big recommendations that I've been hawking for years, neither of which will be for everyone. But it's worth knowing about them. Although I've written extensively about these "prescriptions" in the past, they bear repeating with the latest science.

Aspirin: The Ancient, First Wonder Drug[17]

Aspirin, or acetylsalicylic acid, was developed more than a century ago by the German chemist Felix Hoffmann. It has long proved its value as an analgesic, and now it's earned a label as a potent anti-inflammatory and anticancer drug as well. Two millennia before Hoffmann isolated the compound in a lab, Hippocrates extracted its active ingredient from the bark and leaves of the willow tree to help alleviate pain and fevers.

In 2009, the United States Preventive Services Task Force spoke strongly on the topic of aspirin when it urged men ages forty-five to seventy-nine, and women ages fifty-five to seventy-nine, to take a low-dose aspirin pill daily. The only exceptions to this "rule" would be for those who are already at higher risk for gastrointestinal bleeding or who have certain other health issues. This recommendation was prompted by many high-quality research studies that showed aspirin can substantially reduce the risk of cardiovascular disease, the country's leading killer. Its heart-friendly powers likely entail a variety of mechanisms, including keeping blood clots from forming and dampening inflammation.

Newer reports about aspirin's anticancer qualities have been equally as inspiring. In 2011, British researchers analyzed data from eight long-term studies involving some 25,000 patients and calculated that a small, 75-milligram dose taken daily for at least five years reduced the risk of dying from common cancers by 21 percent.[18] In 2012, The Lancet published two more papers in favor of a daily baby aspirin. The first, reviewing five long-term studies and more than 17,000 patients, found that this ancient drug lowered the risk of getting adenocarcinomas—common malignant cancers that develop in the lungs, colon, and prostate—by an average of 46 percent.[19]

In the second study, researchers led by a group at Oxford analyzed fifty-one different studies comparing patients who took aspirin with those who didn't.[20] The risk of dying from cancer was reduced by 37 percent among those taking aspirin for at least five years. In a smaller section of the study group, three years of daily aspirin use lowered the risk of developing cancer by almost 25 percent when compared with the aspirin-free control group. And in 2015, Harvard researchers calculated a 20 percent lower risk of cancers of the gastrointestinal tract, especially in the colon and rectum, among people taking aspirin.[21] For their study, the researchers collected data on 82,600 women enrolled in the Nurses'

Health Study in 1980 and 47,650 men enrolled in the Health Professionals Follow up Study in 1986. The data included aspirin use, risk factors for cancer, and diagnoses of cancer.

After up to thirty-two years of follow-up, about 20,400 women and 7,570 men developed cancer. Prostate cancer was excluded among the men. The people who took a regular, 325-milligram dose of aspirin at least twice a week enjoyed a lower risk of cancer overall than people who did not take aspirin regularly. This reduced risk was largely due to fewer cases of gastrointestinal cancers, including esophageal cancer, colon cancer, and rectal cancer. Aspirin's anticancer benefits appeared to be related to how much one took: more aspirin, less risk. Amounts in this group of people ranged from less than one aspirin a week to fifteen or more. To gain the most benefit from aspirin meant taking it for at least sixteen years, and the benefit vanished within four years of stopping it.

For some men over the age of forty-five and women over fifty-five, the risks of taking aspirin outweigh any benefits, so you should talk with your doctors before taking a daily dose. My hope is that in the near future we'll develop a new generation of aspirin that eliminates its negative side effects so everyone can benefit from this wonder drug.

Statins: The New, Cheap Wonder Drug

Statins have a negative image in alternative medicine circles that is hard to shake. Statins are compounds that inhibit a liver enzyme that plays a central role in the production of cholesterol. For a long time, we thought the purpose of statins was solely to lower heart disease risk, by virtue of their impact on cholesterol production. But the story doesn't end there. It turns out that they have a profound effect on the entire body, because they help control systemic inflammation—the biological process that can go into overdrive and trigger all kinds of dysfunction and illnesses if left unchecked. Studies in the past decade show that statins can reduce the risk of first-time heart attacks, strokes, and even death from heart disease by about 25 percent to 35 percent (and in many of these people, high cholesterol is not a problem). Studies have also shown that statins can reduce the chances of recurrent strokes or heart attacks by about 40 percent.

In 2012, the *New England Journal of Medicine* published a study involving 300,000 people that indicated a dramatically lowered risk of death from cancer among those who took statins.[22] Such results, among others, encouraged the American College of Cardiology and the American Heart Association to publish new guidelines in 2013, recommending that doctors prescribe statins to patients even if they are at low risk of having a heart attack or stroke. The new guidelines also suggest that doctors *not* put people on statins based on cholesterol levels alone.

The updated guidelines startled and confused doctors, including cardiologists who'd been trained for years to use statins to reduce the risk of cardiovascular events based on cholesterol values alone. It also didn't help that the new online calculator meant to help doctors determine a patient's suitability for cholesterol treatment was called out as being seriously flawed—doubling the estimated risk of heart attack or stroke for the average patient. Not only is the calculator based on outdated and obsolete data, but it—like many other calculators used in medicine—is based on a mathematical model that assumes that risk rises in a straight line. As levels of blood pressure rise, for example, the chances of a heart attack or stroke rise in concert. In reality, though, that line is far from straight. But this calculator is still in use by doctors until a better one emerges. Which is why the conversation about risk factors and the decision to take or not take statins is all the more important to have with your doctors—no matter what any calculator says. Conversation will trump calculation any day.

But the real issue here isn't so much the power of statins on any single pathway in the body that does or does not lead to vascular disease. It's the power they have on the body as a complex system. And to grasp this power, consider their impact on a disease as complex as cancer:

⊙ In the 2012 study I just mentioned, Danish researchers examined whether statin use, started before a cancer diagnosis, was associated with reduced cancer-related death. They assessed death rates among patients from the entire Danish population who had received a diagnosis of cancer between 1995 and 2007, with follow-up until December 31, 2009. Of patients forty years of age or older, 18,721 had used statins regularly before the cancer diagnosis and 277,204 had never used statins. The results? Statin users had a 15 percent lower risk of dying from any cause or from cancer. The reduced cancer-related death among statin users was observed for each of thirteen cancer types.

⊚ A 2015 study looking at roughly 14,000 British lung cancer patients diagnosed between 1998 and 2009 found that those who took statins for a year before getting diagnosed with lung cancer had a 12 percent lower risk of dying from that cancer.[23]

⊚ Another 2015 study examining data from the United Kingdom's Clinical Practice Research Datalink found that statin use was associated with about a 50 percent decreased risk for liver cancer, and this was true whether or not patients had risk factors such as liver disease or diabetes.[24]

⊚ Statin use in men with prostate cancer has been shown to improve their prognosis and slow down the progression of the disease, especially among those who are also taking medication to reduce their levels of male hormones that stimulate their type of cancer.[25] And this likely is related to cholesterol. The body produces male hormones from cholesterol. So by reducing cholesterol levels, statins might cause a reduction in available hormones by inadvertently robbing the body of a key building block for those hormones. What's more, statins might interfere with the process through which prostate tumor cells absorb male hormones. Laboratory tests have shown that statins tend to crowd out hormones, beating them in line to be absorbed by prostate cancer cells.

- A 2014 UK study found that statins may boost colorectal cancer survival. In the largest project to date studying statin use by patients with colorectal cancer, the study combed through the records of more than 7,600 people who'd recently been diagnosed with colorectal cancer.[26] Some people's cancer had spread to nearby lymph nodes. The researchers had, on average, five years' worth of patient history, including prescription records and death records. From 1998 to 2009, the study period, nearly 1,650 patients died of colorectal cancer. For those who took statin drugs for more than a year, their risk of dying from their colon cancer shrank 36 percent. People who used statins for less than one year reduced their risk by 21 percent. Overall, the study concluded that statin use was associated with a 29 percent decrease in the odds of dying from cancer. The study also documented a 25 percent lower risk of death *from any cause* among those who took statins.

- In a 2013 nationwide Finnish study, statin use was associated with a 66 percent reduction in the risk of dying from breast cancer.[27] The researchers looked at statin use and breast cancer mortality among the 31,114 women with breast cancer who were diagnosed in Finland between 1995 and 2003. During follow-up, 6,011 of the women died, 3,169 due to breast cancer. The death rate among statin users was 7.5 percent while among non–statin users it was 21 percent.

I will also add that in 2015, a new report published in the *Journal of the American Medical Association* confirmed that the latest guidelines are actually more accurate and efficient than ever before, despite the initial reactions among doctors who were used to looking at just cholesterol levels.[28] Approximately 10 million US adults are newly eligible for statin therapy under the new guidelines, and it's estimated that between 41,000 and 63,000 cardiovascular events—heart attacks, strokes, or deaths from cardiovascular disease—could be prevented over a ten-year period. The *JAMA* report points out that the 2013 guidelines accomplish three important tasks: they broaden prevention efforts to encompass all forms of heart disease; they identify adults at high risk for cardiovascular trouble who could benefit from statins; and they distinguish low-risk patients who do not need to take the drugs.

Statins do have their opponents. You'll find articles and studies linking statin use with *increased* risk of cancer and death. Some implicate them in upping the risk for dementia and type 2 diabetes. But therein lies the challenge: identifying the relevant facts and details, and weighing risks and benefits smartly. In the case of the widely publicized study that showed a relationship between statin use and the development of type 2 diabetes, for example, there was no data regarding weight, ethnicity, and family history—all important risk factors for the development of diabetes.

Keep in mind that, with regard to many of these studies that show a drop in the risk of an illness or death, there are any number of other differences between people who take statins and those who don't that might explain the outcome, rather than statin use itself. None of these studies—even the ones that condemn statins—can prove a cause-and-effect link. They can speak only to an association. And that's why they should be considered on a case-by-case basis in the context of the individual, as with everything else in medicine.

Unfortunately, statins are often seen as the prime example of all that is wrong with Big Pharma. They are criticized as overpriced, overmarketed, and overprescribed, while their risks are underplayed. But a ninety-day supply of a statin at Walmart, without health insurance, costs only $10! And, most of all, we cannot ignore the data showing their power. Are statins for everyone? Of course not. But they should be in the conversation.

Earlier I noted how we may have all the drugs we'll ever need to prevent and fight disease. When it comes to statins, for example, it just may be that their effects on the body can address a surprising number of maladies, including infections as grave and fierce as Ebola.

More than ten years ago, doctors noted striking similarities between people infected with the Ebola virus and those with bacterial sepsis, an uncontrolled bacterial infection in the blood. Both diseases involve a major dysfunction of the cells that line blood vessels throughout the body, which can lead to severe abnormalities in blood coagulation. The result can be weakness or failure of internal organs, primarily the liver and kidneys, and death is a real possibility. A similar event occurs in people with other types of acute critical illness, such as influenza and pneumonia.

Ebola has a high mortality rate, and especially since the outbreak that swept through Western Africa in 2014 and traveled to America via a few people infected with the virus, scientists have been on a hunt for effective treatments. And they've been thinking outside the box in their search for drugs that are relatively easy to access and inexpensive. Enter the possibility of statins, which are among the drugs that can modify or reverse the abnormalities of endothelial function and coagulation. A clinical trial published in the journal *Critical Care* in 2012 showed that early treatment of sepsis patients with a statin decreased the occurrence of organ failure by 83 percent.[29] This is the same complication that often kills people who've contracted Ebola.

So could statins and other immunomodulatory drugs similarly prevent organ failure in Ebola patients and spare their lives? Future research will figure this out. While these drugs can't prevent infection itself, if they can prevent potentially fatal complications like organ failure, they will likely be part of the treatment protocol until an effective preventive measure such as a vaccine against the virus can be developed.

Once again, this goes to show the power of what's already in our arsenal. The Lucky Years are already here. And even though we're entering a high-tech era of medicine, the same old ancient secrets to a good, long life are still relevant. Nothing will ever be able to substitute for things like sleep, sex, and touch—and perhaps gnawing on the bark of a willow tree.

CHAPTER 9

The Butterfly Effect

Get Ready to Flap Your Wings

All religions, arts, and sciences are branches of the same tree. All these aspirations are directed toward ennobling man's life, lifting it from the sphere of mere physical existence, and leading the individual toward freedom.

—Albert Einstein

Medicine is a science of uncertainty and an art of probability.

—Sir William Osler

If a jeweler tried to sell you a diamond that looked fake, you'd probably find another jeweler because something in your gut would tell you to move on. If you've ever bought a car, you likely used your intuition at some point to know which one would be right for you, walking away from candidates you simply had bad feelings about. And if your doctor told you at your next appointment that you need major surgery to remove a mysterious lump in your side, you'd seek a second opinion as soon as possible—not because you don't trust your doctor, but because your instinct says that's the best thing to do, period.

Throughout this book, I've highlighted the value that technologies will bring to medicine. But along the way I've also underscored the power of insight that cannot be quantified by a device, app, medical test, or other technology. Most of us do have an inherent sense of what's good for us, much in the same way we know the difference between right and wrong. I'm not one to use absolutes that much, but I'm absolutely sure that there will always be an element of art in the practice and execution of medicine no matter how techy we get. And as patients and consumers, we'll also have to employ a little bit of artful intuition and science in our lives to benefit from any technology. I can't reiterate the following enough: there's nothing more powerful than the decidedly unscientific and unadulterated question from doctor to patient, "How do you feel?"

All the technology in the world can't give you that answer; it must come from a part of you that's untouchable. When I send patients home with a recommended strategy for their treatment plan, I don't only want to be able to cure them, which isn't possible in many cases. I want to make them feel better and live better. I also want them to be comfortable with the decisions they're making about their health, decisions that stem from science but are couched within their value systems. After all, what matters in life anymore if we can't feel good and secure?

In this final chapter, I'm going to touch upon a few notes that drive home important points for entering the Lucky Years. At the heart of this message will be the omnipotence of your own intuition and gut instinct as you venture into the Lucky Years. The achievement of wellness is an art, not a true science, that is practiced jointly by you and your physician.

Hunch Power

In a widely referenced anecdote, a panel of art experts is brought together to sniff out phony works of art. They are invited into a room where ten or so paintings are on display, each allegedly the work of the famous Renaissance artist Rembrandt—but some are by imitators. It takes these experts mere seconds to identify the fakes from the real ones. When asked how they can come to their conclusions so quickly, and what makes the forgeries so obviously counterfeit, they cannot articulate their reasoning other than to say something along the lines of "I just know" or "I can *see* it." And it turns out that their hunches are accurate.

This phenomenon is the core theme in Malcolm Gladwell's 2005 book *Blink: The Power of Thinking Without Thinking*,[1] in which he writes:

> We live in a world that assumes that the quality of a decision is directly related to the time and effort that went into making it. When doctors are faced with a difficult diagnosis, they order more tests, and when we are uncertain about what we hear, we ask for a second opinion. And what do we tell our children? Haste makes waste. Look before you leap. Stop and *think*. Don't judge a book by its cover. We believe that we are always better off gathering as much information as possible and spending as much time as possible in deliberation. We only trust conscious decision making. But there are moments, particularly in times of stress, when haste does not make waste, when our snap judgments and first impressions can offer a much better means of making sense of the world. The first task of *Blink* is to convince you of a simple fact: decisions made very quickly can be every bit as good as decisions made cautiously and deliberately.[2]

Gladwell opens the book with a story about a fake kouros, a sixth-century BC Greek statue of a larger-than-life-size nude youth carved from marble.

In the 1980s, the J. Paul Getty Museum paid around $9 million to acquire one of only twelve kouroi left in the world. It was hailed as one of the most important works of ancient art to enter the United States since World War II. Despite some initial suspicions among museum

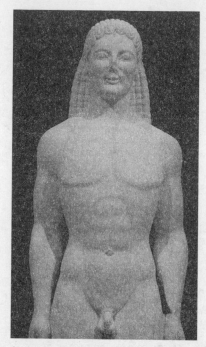

A photo of the infamous Getty kouros. The marble sculpture was purchased by the J. Paul Getty Museum in 1985 for $9 million.

officials, the Getty decided to purchase the statue after an exhaustive investigation that lasted more than a year. The probe included testing the statue's age, consulting sculpture experts in Athens, and background checks into the documentation of the statue's former owners. In the end, scientists and lawyers hired by the Getty said it was not a fake. In October 1986, satisfied that the kouros was an original, the Getty put it on display. Unfortunately, once the sculpture went up for viewing, longtime art experts took one glance at it and thought it was bogus. The first person to doubt its authenticity was an Italian art historian, Federico Zeri, who said that the statue's fingernails "seemed wrong to him." He could not express exactly why they looked wrong, but he had a bad feeling about it based on having seen many similar objects that were real.

When several other art experts experienced the same doubts, the Getty commenced further inquiry into the sculpture's origin. Much to the Getty's dismay, the possibility that it was a reproduction became impossible to escape. More research revealed that parts of the sculpture fit into different time periods, and it was determined that a good forgery could pass a core sample test if the statue were soaked in potato mold. The beleaguered statue remains on display today, but its placard reads: "About 530 BC, or modern forgery." Despite all the technology in the world, neither art historians nor scientists have ever been able to resolve the issue of the kouros's authenticity completely. The Getty's curator of antiquities at the height of the controversy, Marion True, believed in the work's authenticity at first but then conceded: "Science isn't the final word. It is flexible and changeable as new evidence becomes available, and as new technology is brought to the question at hand."[3] How true that statement is, especially in the realm of health and medicine.

Gladwell's book is largely about "rapid cognition," or first impressions and instant decisions—and how science and culture don't appreciate the importance of immediate reactions as much as slower, more deliberate decision processes.

Each of us has the ability to come to snap conclusions. It's built into our survival mechanisms. In life-threatening situations, we need to be able to make quick decisions based on the available information. A lot of our functioning in fact happens without us having to think consciously. Throughout the day, our brain toggles back and forth between conscious and unconscious thought. It's as if we have two brains. We have one brain for carefully analyzing and categorizing, and another that can size things up intuitively first and address questions later. Gladwell introduces the concept of "thin-slicing," which is "the ability of our unconscious to find patterns in situations and behavior based on very narrow slices of experience." By identifying an underlying pattern, we can even "read" and evaluate complex situations. Which is how art experts can often assess the authenticity of a work of art in an instant, getting an actual physical feeling as they look at a sculpture or painting. Something in their gut tells them this is the real thing or a rip-off.

The reason I'm sharing all this detail about spurious art and the experts who argue over what they see is that the subject of objectivity and artistry—and pattern recognition—is relevant in health. We all establish patterns of behavior, or habits, that play into our health and the path that our health takes. And we all have hunch power: the ability to know instinctively what we should be doing to lead healthy, strong lives. These two characteristics—habits and intuition—are ultimately what make us human and will allow us to capitalize on the Lucky Years. As we encounter a wealth of data and technologies to help us understand our individual contexts, we'll be equipped to take control of our health like never before, shape new habits, gain better intuition, and be well prepared for what the future holds.

More than 40 percent of the actions we perform each day are not actual decisions—they are habits.[4] So if habits command much of our daily lives, then in the Lucky Years we need to tap our intuition continually, and change ingrained habits, as we encounter new information and have access to technologies that can better our lives. If we stay stuck in old habits that don't work for us anymore, or worse, harm us, then we won't be able to enjoy the Lucky Years and all that they can offer.

As we grow older, many habits become background noise that we ignore, and unfortunately, this can have unintended consequences when we end up with a chronic condition we could have prevented. Those who notice and try to stay exceptionally attuned to their habits—ushering in the ones that support wellness and doing away with those that don't—are typically the ones who stay healthier. The fifty-year-old who looks ten to fifteen years younger and has the heart and brain of a thirty-year-old is the person who has made slight shifts in her habits as time went on. The eighty-year-old who can still live independently and play with his grandchildren has similarly adjusted his habits through the years. These people have honed what's called their perceptual intuition skills, something we'd all do well to develop.

Malcolm Gladwell isn't the only one who has popularized the concept of "thinking without thinking." Perceptual intuition is a popular field of study currently gaining momentum in psychological, educational, and scientific circles, and it's a powerful factor in achieving better health.[5] I've already been describing perceptual intuition, which in the simplest terms means being able to use your gut instinct to solve problems and "perceive" certain things. People with well-developed perceptual intuition skills—such as the baseball player who can visualize pitches early, the art collector who can instantly spot a counterfeit painting, the doctor who can look at a patient and know something is wrong—have a great "third eye." This inner source of intuitive wisdom helps them make quick and, in many cases, accurate or correct decisions.

When you think about it, perceptual intuition is a way of looking at yourself and asking, "How can I live better tomorrow based on what I'm doing today? What habits do I need to change based on what I know? What new technologies or habits should I bring into my life?"

Although we're not always aware of it, we ask ourselves these questions every single day, many times over. Whenever we're faced with a decision, from deciding what to eat to which medication to try to treat a condition, our first questions are always "What are the options? What are the facts and what data are available to me? What should my solution or outcome be?" All of this activity that our brain performs, below our conscious radar, is a perfect example of our perceptions at work helping us to solve problems and make good decisions. I encourage you to tap your intuition as much as possible and bring more consciousness to those important decisions in life that relate with your health. Identify the phony from the real in health advice and know that your choices must reflect *you*—your biology, your context, and your values. And then let science—and the art you and your doctor bring to it—do the rest.

A Rough Look

In the world of medicine, a new concept is being used, stolen from physics and photography, that will increasingly help us in the Lucky Years. Because many times we can't understand everything, scientists are *coarse graining* biology to make models to predict outcomes. Coarse graining comes originally from photography: as you twist the focus on the lens, you go more and more out of focus until all you can see when you point the camera at a friend is the outline of a human.

If you turn the lens the other way and get into better focus, more and more details come to you—what your friend is wearing, the expression on her face, and her hairstyle. But you didn't need any of that to know it was a human being. Sometimes we in medicine look at way too many details and try to put them into a model, when if we'd take a step back and examine a coarse-grained element instead, it would work much better. This is not unlike the art historian who can look at a paint-

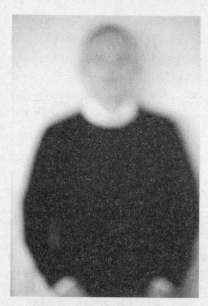

A coarse-grained image of me. The details of my face and body are obscured, but you can still tell the photograph is of a human.

ing from far away and tell if it's real or not without having to conduct any fancy scientific research on the canvas or examine it up close with a magnifying glass.

The physics and climate-modeling worlds have learned so much by taking this approach. The meteorologist doesn't go thousands of feet up in the sky every day and measure wind speed, temperature, and moisture to help predict the weather. Instead, he looks at the shape of the clouds as a coarse-grained element of everything going on, and uses this to help model the forecast. Medicine has to go the same way. If I want to know if you are stressed, I can measure your adrenal and neurohormones and study your brain activity with a functional MRI (magnetic resonance imaging) or PET (positron-emission tomography) scan, or I can simply measure your heart rate variability (HRV)—the time intervals between heartbeats, which aren't always the same.

Broadly speaking, coarse graining means being able to look at a complex system or structure and make a rough sketch of it without all the nitty-gritty details. This coarse-grained element can then be used as a surrogate for all of the nitty-gritty details that either can't be measured efficiently or can't be measured at all. Many of the technologies that will dominate in the Lucky Years will help us coarse grain biology around a specific outcome. For example, we will measure your skin's electrical conductivity (termed either galvanic skin response, GSR, or electrodermal response) between two points on your arm as a way of measuring that your body is excited or tiring. It sounds pretty wild, but the skin momentarily becomes a better conductor of electricity when external or internal stimuli occur. I could use this technology to understand which songs on the radio "charge you up" while you are driving, and the car could play these particular tunes if it senses you are about to fall asleep at the wheel.

On a similar note, consider my friend who called me a few weeks ago with an exciting story to tell. He had been wearing a device that gives him a readout through the day of his heart rate. He had a baseline heart rate in the high 50s, but noted that his heart rate went up to the mid-60s on one particular day. And then he came down with a virus. This observation—seeing the trend in his heart rate change and culminate in getting sick—thrilled him. Having this kind of knowledge in advance is increasingly going to happen in the Lucky Years, allowing us to better prepare for or perhaps totally evade those times when we're destined to be under the weather.

Here are a few more examples: the size of your red blood cells will be used as a coarse-grained measure to check for iron deficiency instead of measuring blood iron and its partners. Cells deficient in iron are much smaller than their counterparts with iron. The "how do you feel" question will be employed with advanced cancer after starting a new treatment to determine if a therapy is working rather than just measuring all of the tumors in the body. While such a broad, general question may sound "unscientific," it can lead to real solutions and useful information to effect better outcomes. New technologies will be used to further coarse-grain biology and give us shortcuts to help answer some of the key questions that dominate in medicine. Can we coarse grain aging? Aging is a gradual deterioration of organ systems in the body. If we could measure it, doctors could start clinical trials to slow the process, starting at a young age. But it's likely the subjects would outlive the researchers, using our current standard of survival as the endpoint of clinical trials. That is not a tenable solution. We have to develop coarse-grained measures of aging and use these as surrogates, or representatives, for survival. For example, maybe a combination of how you look, how you feel, and other coarse-grained elements can be combined with measurements of organ function to yield one number. This number could be studied in clinical trials as a proxy for "biological age." The comparison of biological age to chronological age would be the endpoint for the intervention. Going forward, you and I will be able to decelerate our aging pace using real-time metrics, such as this.

"I Shall . . ."

In 2014, I had the pleasure of spending the weekend in Berlin with Muhammad Yunus, a true hero of epic proportions today from my perspective.[6] I don't know if I've ever met a humbler or more altruistic individual, a man now in his seventies whose passion for helping mankind is surely in his DNA. Yunus has created more than fifty self-sustaining companies to lift his country out of poverty, and he can claim zero ownership in those enterprises. Famous in his native country of Bangladesh and world renowned as a civic leader and successful social entrepreneur and economist, Yunus was awarded the Nobel Peace Prize in 2006 for founding the Grameen Bank and pioneering the practice of microfinance—providing banking to entrepreneurs and small businesses that would not otherwise have access to such services. Some have called him the godfather of microcredit. What started as a passion to help "just one person each day" has grown into a global phenomenon of two hundred fifty microcredit programs in nearly one hundred countries. His story exemplifies not only the power of blending art and science, but also catering to people's basic needs, intuitions, and motivations in pursuit of innovation—and a healthier tomorrow.

Yunus initially got into the business during the famine of 1974, when dying Bangladeshi people began to beg for help from wealthier citizens in the city of Dhaka. Watching this tragedy as an economics professor at Chittagong University, Yunus grew frustrated. His lofty economic theories were not doing anything to help his fellow Bangladeshi families who were barely surviving. He then began to take his discontent to the streets, speaking with the poor and thinking about how he could help them. At first, he lent twenty-seven dollars to a group of forty-two people in a nearby village who were being victimized by shady, unethical lenders. This inspired the idea of lending small amounts of money to impoverished individuals who could then work toward giving back somehow through a trade or craft, essentially starting businesses that would support their livelihood and contribute to society at large. Yunus couldn't get local banks to participate in the lending, however. So he vowed to do it himself, and Grameen Bank was born in 1976.

Yunus taught me a lot about how to think about and approach health that weekend in Berlin. Even though he's a man of the banking world, he's also a man of the public health world, always innovating ways to bring the two together to effect change in his society. Bangladesh is among the most densely populated countries in the world with more than 160 million people living in an area the size of Iowa. Although it has made significant strides in human and social development since declaring its independence in 1971, Bangladesh has faced numerous political, economic, social, and environmental challenges, including political instability, corruption, and immense poverty. Enter Yunus and his ideas based on a simple concept: "Lend poor people money on terms that are suitable to them, teach them a few sound financial principles, and they will help themselves."

One of Yunus's most prized legacies is how he transformed the lending industry in Bangladesh in response to local loan sharking. Proving that the poor can be reliable borrowers (despite conventional banking dogma), his bank has disbursed billions of dollars to millions of borrowers who have no collateral, and it has a 98 percent payback rate even though there's no legal instrument or written contract involved. Most of his borrowers have risen out of acute poverty and almost all are women. In fact, 98 percent of his loan recipients are women who meet once a week and, through incentives, help to ensure their individual loan repayments. Why focus on lending women money? Traditionally, in the third world, men are the recipients of loans from banks. But this is where Yunus was brilliant: not only were women more responsible about repaying the loans and families benefited more when the women controlled the money, but he also knew that the women in Bangladesh controlled health decisions in their families. So by focusing on them, he could revolutionize health in his country. And he did.

In 1984, Grameen finalized its "16 Decisions," essentially a set of commandments that every borrower must accept. The bank set a high bar for itself, with the goal of making each of its branches free of poverty as defined by benchmarks such as having adequate food and access to clean water and latrines. Among the Decisions stipulated in his loans:

> Decision Four: "We shall grow vegetables all the year round. We shall eat plenty of them and sell the surplus."
> Decision Nine: "We shall build and use pit latrines."

When I asked Yunus about the latrine commitment, he explained how sanitation in Bangladesh was horrible at the time his bank started thriving. The widespread squalor led to outbreaks of cholera. People were relieving themselves outside in the open air, allowing the disease to spread. This motivated him to put a condition on the loans that you had to dig a toilet hole in order to get the money. "A pit latrine is a simple, practical way of drastically reducing the incidence of diseases spread by contact with human waste," he told me. His bankers would actually go into the countryside where their customers were and check for the latrines before dispensing the money.

The incidence of cholera started to plummet. In fact, the wealthy women who didn't need loans were getting jealous that the poor had pit latrines close to their tents. In Islam, the women don't regularly go out in daylight, so they'd have to wait (uncomfortably so) until night fell, then walk to the outskirts of the village to go to the bathroom outside. Soon everyone was building his or her own pit latrines.

Yunus continued to take his ideas further. His bank staff taught its members how to prepare a saline solution at home to fight dehydration due to cholera. They developed a rhyming poem so everyone would remember the basic home ingredients to put into water to make the electrolyte solution. Yunus also founded a social company to build and distribute toilets. To further fight malnutrition, in 2007 Yunus partnered with Dannon, the French multinational milk product company, to develop an inexpensive, fortified yogurt chock full of all required nutrients. Grameen Danone sought to sell cheaply and it took no profit. It has been very successful.

For another example of Yunus's genius, he once noted that when he would visit villages at night, the children couldn't read. They were suffering from night blindness, a common result of severe vitamin A deficiency. So he sprinted into action again, this time organizing a business to distribute vitamin A–rich vegetable seeds—for a penny a pack. He first looked into starting a vitamin company, but people didn't want to take pills. If he didn't charge, the people would perceive no value. So he solved the problem with the penny-a-pack seeds that would supply the vitamin A naturally (hence Decision Four). The business flourished until soon he was the largest seed supplier in Bangladesh and, not surprisingly, children could see again at night.

In 2011, Yunus addressed the uneven doctor-to-nurse ratio (3:1) by starting a nursing college funded by a for-profit social business that's poised to break even in 2016. Once the $6 million initial funding for the school is paid back, he'll go on to build another nursing school and another. The qualification, however, to enter this nursing program is that your mother must be a Grameen Bank borrower. The bank gives the loan to these women who get accepted to the nursing college. They pay it off slowly over their career through salary deductions. And they are guaranteed a job at graduation, which psychologically helps.

I could go on and on about all the innovative things Yunus has done to transform his community—and the world at large. He is the kind of visionary we need today. He has set a terrific example of how we can incentivize people to be accountable for their health and wellness. He's created a system for turning hope into real, concrete possibilities. I love how he encapsulates his mission: "It's not about money; it is about creative ideas." And I'll add ". . . that can change the world." I also couldn't agree more with his belief that "Charity is not the answer to poverty."

In America, we love incentives. But we also love our entitlements. A question we must all ask is, who or what is driving us to prevent disease? Sometimes we get such incentives from our children, the wish to conquer a diagnosis, or the mere desire to feel and look better than we do. But it's hard to inspire people to do something today that will affect them a decade later. There's just no feedback loop in the health domain; you're not paid to stay at a healthy weight or avoid artificial sweeteners; you don't get tax credits for exercising at least three times a week; and you don't get an extra week of paid vacation if you show that you're engaged in activities that lower your stress levels and keep you happy.

So where does that leave us? Having to create our own incentives— finishing the "I shall . . ." statement by making commitments to ourselves. And that process begins by knowing who you are and, perhaps more important, *how you feel*.

Flap Your Wings

For every intervention you adopt, you create change. This was articulated beautifully by the late Edward Lorenz: when a butterfly flutters its wings in one part of the world, it can eventually cause a hurricane in another. Lorenz was an MIT meteorologist who tried to explain why it is so hard to make good weather forecasts; he wound up starting a scientific revolution called chaos theory. In the early 1960s, he noticed that small differences in a dynamic system such as the atmosphere could give rise to vast and often unexpected results. These observations ultimately led him to develop what became known as the butterfly effect, a term that grew out of an academic paper he presented in 1972 entitled "Predictability: Does the Flap of a Butterfly's Wings in Brazil Set Off a Tornado in Texas?"[7]

The butterfly effect has significant relevance in all matters of health. We are each agents of change in the Lucky Years; we are each butterflies flapping our wings in a space-time continuum on earth. How we live today affects how we are tomorrow. It also impacts the people with whom we interact, our neighbors, the next generation, our children, and their children. It's easy to cast blame on big business, insurance companies, and the weaknesses in our national health care policies. It's much harder to point the finger at citizens and ask for help in creating change. But we must empower people to take charge of their health in ways they haven't before if we're ever going to rise above our challenges. The conversation in Washington circles continues to revolve around issues with health insurance policies and health care finance while ducking the most essential policy of all—the one each of us makes with ourselves. We need to be encouraged to sign personal policies that specify the things we will do to support our health and bring down our risks for an early death. And those personal policies are priceless.

In addition to creating our own personal policy to thrive in the Lucky Years, it behooves us to lobby our political leaders to push the idea that prevention is the cure. We all love a good cure. We like watching our government spend money on discovering a remedy for a serious disease, but now that we've knocked out a lot of maladies that once factored into our mortality (e.g., smallpox, polio, mumps, rubella), we need to spend more money researching and combating chronic illnesses that usually can be prevented—from diabetes to cancer. Lately, Congress has funneled more money toward understanding diseases and potential treatments at the expense of focusing on prevention. If we have therapies that work to prevent various illnesses, why don't we promote those? Here's a thought: California's tobacco control program cost $2.4 billion to run between 1989 and 2008, but resulted in health expenditure savings of $134 billion (and more important, saved countless lives).[8] A very small percentage of our federal money is spent on antitobacco campaigns. In 2012, tobacco companies spent $9.6 billion marketing cigarettes and smokeless tobacco in the United States alone. This amount translates to about $26 million *daily*, or more than $1 million *every hour*.[9] Nineteen percent of high schoolers are still smoking today.[10] That's 19 percent too many.

In preparing to write this book, I asked a few friends and colleagues what they'd do differently if they could write a letter to their much younger selves. All of them wished they'd avoided the conditions they grapple with today. They would have told their younger selves to establish better habits sooner and to have the foresight to know what was coming down the pipeline in their health life. Granted, most of us would love a glimpse into our future and future health. That's not possible. But prevention is, and it's especially possible in the Lucky Years. When we were young, we planned our educations, careers, and even our retirements. We didn't plan our future health. Now that we can more easily do that, it's imperative. It's essential. And all that's asked of us is that we start to flap our wings.

As the Savage in Huxley's *Brave New World* says, "All right then . . . I'm claiming the right to be unhappy. Not to mention the right to grow old and ugly and impotent; the right to have syphilis and cancer; the right to have too little to eat; the right to be lousy; the right to live in constant apprehension of what may happen tomorrow; the right to catch typhoid; the right to be tortured by unspeakable pains of every kind."[11] After that statement comes a long silence, and then the Savage says, "I claim them all."

The Lucky Years are here and we all must adapt to take advantage. As the Savage says, it is our right to do nothing, but we also have the ability, the technology, and the wisdom to do the opposite. And that requires action. I imagine the last person to buy the older model of a smartphone days before the surprise launch of the new model feels buyer's remorse every time he sees a friend with the new one. A friend called me recently to discuss getting an elective surgical procedure to correct one of the changes that happens with aging. In discussing with him whether this made sense or not (for the record, I was against the procedure), I told him that in the near future we may be able to awaken his own quiescent stem cells and allow him to go back in time, but having the surgical procedure now may preclude this. His sentiment quickly changed. He put his faith in the Lucky Years rather than resort to a temporary fix. I hope by focusing on prevention today, there will be no remorse and we can all benefit and enjoy what the Lucky Years have to offer.

Acknowledgments

I thank my patients for allowing me to be involved with their care and their lives. They demonstrate to me daily how the Lucky Years are benefiting all of us. At the same time, I continually realize that the current progress isn't enough. We still need more advances to alleviate suffering, but I am more confident and optimistic than ever that the breakthroughs will arrive.

It is not just a privilege, but it is also a responsibility to strive to educate about health. I have never been on this path alone and have many to thank. This book reflects the culmination of not just my lifetime work in science and medicine, but also my ongoing collaboration with many individuals and teams of people. First, I thank my collaborator Kristin Loberg. Kristin and I have been working together for six years now, and I still get excited every time we speak. She is an amazing partner, an insightful thinker, a remarkably talented writer, and a good friend. I would like to thank her family, Lawrence, Colin, and Teddy, for allowing me to spend the precious time with her over the past years.

To Robert Barnett, who has expertly and caringly represented, protected, and guided me through this process. Your mentorship, friendship, and wisdom have meant so much to me. David Povich, thank you for being a guiding light to me. You have both been extraordinary in looking after me.

I have been with the same publishing house for the three books I have written, and I couldn't imagine a better and more supportive environment. I wish to thank the crew at Simon & Schuster, led by Priscilla Painton, whose support, faith, and skill made this book possible. I can easily state that Priscilla's exquisite editorial leadership made this a much better, clearer, and focused book. Thanks also to her fantastic colleagues, including Marie Florio, Allison Har-zvi, Larry Hughes, Sophia Jimenez, Jessica Chin, Kristen Lemire, Richard Rhorer, Jackie Seow, Dana Trocker, and the fantastic boss Jonathan Karp. Thank you for putting up with me (I know it isn't easy) and your continued support. To Steve Bennett and AuthorBytes, thanks for the creative and dynamic website management.

I am also indebted to my team at the USC Westside Cancer Center and the Center for Applied Molecular Medicine, who enable me to wear multiple hats—to be a physician, teacher, and researcher—and find the time to write. I want to thank particularly my fantastic assistant Wendy Piatt, and former assistant Autumn Beemer, and the clinic team of Olga Castellanos, Shelly Danowsky, Adam Feldman, Angel Jones, Bill Loadvine, Kelly La Mont, Michael Rice, Cindy Richards, Kelly Santoro, Rachel Twomey, Julianne Yu, and Mitchell Gross, all under the inspirational leadership of Lisa Flashner. Thank you for your loyalty and friendship and the caring you give to the patients we are honored to treat. To the research team including lab chief Shannon Mumenthaler, Jonathan Katz, Dan Ruderman, Paul Macklin, Kian Kani, and Yvonne Suarez, and the rest of the dedicated scientists. Thank you for pushing my thinking forward and your work in figuring out better ways to understand and treat disease. To my science mentors, collaborators, and friends Andrea Armani, Anthony Atala, Anna Barker, Paul Davies, Scott Fraser, Sam Gambhir, Murray Gell-Mann, Inderbir Gill, Dana Goldman, Danny Hillis, Cliff Hudis, Carl Kesselman, Parag Mallick, Franziska Michor, Vincent Miller, Larry Norton, Carmen Puliafito, Michael Quick, Chris Rose, Howard Scher, P. K. Shah, Jeff Trent, and Yannis Yortsos.

I have the privilege of seeing the breaking health and technology information daily through my involvement with CBS News. Many of the ideas discussed in *The Lucky Years* originated from stories I initially did with *CBS This Morning*. To the outstanding leadership at CBS News, including Chris Licht, Lulu Chiang, Jon LaPook, and David Rhodes, who empower me to educate and inform; and to Susan Schackman and Leigh Ann Winick who collaborate with me on every story and are excellent at distilling the essence and truth from science news. An extremely difficult task! The anchor team of Gayle King, Norah O'Donnell, and Charlie Rose is an absolute pleasure to talk with at 4:00 a.m. and 5:00 a.m. Los Angeles time. Your collective passion to understand and enlighten comes through every day. I am lucky to be a part of such a program.

To my friends Dominick Anfuso, Marc Benioff, Glenn Boghosian, Yael Braun, Jerry Breslauer, Eli Broad, Sharon Brous, Bill Campbell, Steve, Jean and Stacey Case, Robert Day, Michael Dell, John Doerr, Bryce Duffy, Larry Ellison, Bob Evans, Sandy Gleysteen, Darryl Goldman, Jimmy (Taboo) Gomez, Al Gore, Brad Grey, Davis Guggenheim, Yoshiki Hayashi, Uri Herscher, Walter Isaacson, Peter Jacobs (and the CAA team), Ashton Kutcher, Jimmy Linn, Dan Loeb, Max Nikias, Fabian Oberfeld, Howard Owens, Chemi and Shimon Peres, Amy Powell, Robin Quivers, Bruce Ramer, Linda Ramone, Ed Razek, Shari Redstone, Sumner Redstone, Joe Schoendorf, Dov Seidman, Greg Simon, Bonnie Solow, Steven Spielberg, Tom Staggs, Elle and Paul Stephens, Gregorio Stephenson, Howard Stern, Meir Teper, Yossi Vardi, Jay Walker, David Weissman, Will.i.am, and Neil Young: your mentorship, friendship, and advice are appreciated beyond measure. To my personal exercise team of Heidi Kling, Anne Van Valkenburg, and Nereida Vital, thank you for helping me to practice what I preach.

Lastly, to my family for their unwavering support and love; thank you to my beautiful and inspiring wife, Amy, and our two fantastic children Sydney and Miles, and our goofy and loyal dog, Sadie. To my mother, Sandy, and father, Zalman, who have been role models and inspired me from day one in Baltimore. And to the rest of the Povich and Agus gang, I thank you and love you.

Lastly, to the readers, thank you for believing in *The Lucky Years* . . .

Notes

The following is a list of citations organized by chapter. Included, where appropriate, are notes that you might find helpful in learning more about some of the ideas and concepts expressed in this book. This is by no means an exhaustive list, for each of these citations could be complemented with dozens if not hundreds of others. From a practical standpoint, I was limited on how many studies and references I could include. But this list will help you learn more and live up to the implied lessons and principles of *The Lucky Years*. These materials can also open other doors for further research and inquiry. If a reference that was mentioned in the book is not listed here, please refer to the website, DavidAgus.com, where a more comprehensive list is found.

Introduction: Destiny of the Species

1. Clive M. McCay, Frank Pope, and Wanda Lunsford, "Experimental Prolongation of the Life Span," *Bulletin of the New York Academy of Medicine* 32, no. 2 (1956): 91–101.
2. Note: this research was presented at the 28th Graduate Fortnight on *Problems of Aging* on October 10, 1955, and subsequently published as a *Bulletin of the New York Academy of Medicine* in 1956. (See above citation.)
3. For a review of the history of parabiosis and its long list of references, see Megan Scudellari, "Ageing Research: Blood to Blood," *Nature* 517 (January 22, 2015): 426–29, doi:10.1038/517426a. For a layman's read of the latest studies, check out Ian Sample, "Can We Reverse the Ageing Process by Putting Young Blood into Older People?," *Guardian* (UK), August 4, 2015, www.theguardian.com/science/2015/aug/04/can-we-reverse-ageing-process-young-blood-older-people, accessed August 6, 2015. Also note that today these experiments are conducted carefully to reduce the animals' discomfort and death as much as possible. The mice chosen to

become like Siamese twins are the same gender and roughly the same size. Two weeks before their union, they are socialized with each other, presumably to get to know each other and become comfortable in close proximity. The surgery itself is done in a warm, sterile environment with anesthesia and antibiotics to prevent infection. Once joined, the mice act normally: eating, drinking, and doing their usual things. Should they need to be separated, this can be accomplished easily. Although the procedure has been done on frogs, insects, and small freshwater invertebrates called hydra, it works best in rodents because they recover well from the surgery.

4. Wanda Ruth Lunsford, "Parabiosis as a Method for Studying Factors Which Affect Aging in Rats" (master's thesis, Cornell University, September 1960).

5. F. C. Ludwig and R. M. Elashoff, "Mortality in Syngeneic Rat Parabionts of Different Chronological Age," *Transactions of the New York Academy of Sciences* 34 (1972): 582–87.

6. D. E. Wright et al., "Physiological Migration of Hematopoietic Stem and Progenitor Cells," *Science* 294 (2001): 1933–36.

7. A. J. Wagers et al., "Little Evidence for Developmental Plasticity of Adult Hematopoietic Stem Cells," *Science* 297 (2002): 2256–59.

8. S. A. Villeda et al., "Young Blood Reverses Age-Related Impairments in Cognitive Function and Synaptic Plasticity in Mice," *Nature Medicine* 20, no. 6 (June 2014): 659–63, doi:10.1038/nm.3569, Epub May 4, 2014.

9. L. Katsimpardi et al., "Vascular and Neurogenic Rejuvenation of the Aging Mouse Brain by Young Systemic Factors," *Science* 344 (2014): 630–34.

10. F. Demontis et al., "Intertissue Control of the Nucleolus Via a Myokine-Dependent Longevity Pathway," *Cell Reports* 7, no. 5 (June 12, 2014): 1481–94.

11. C. Elabd et al., "Oxytocin Is an Age-Specific Circulating Hormone That Is Necessary for Muscle Maintenance and Regeneration," *Nature Communications* 5 (June 10, 2014): 4082.

12. G. S. Baht et al., "Exposure to a Youthful Circulation Rejuvenates Bone Repair Through Modulation of β-catenin," *Nature Communications* 6 (May 2015): 7131, doi:10.1038/ncomms8131.

13. Andy Grove, *Only the Paranoid Survive* (New York: Doubleday Business, 1996).

14. H. L. Rehm et al., "ClinGen—the Clinical Genome Resource," *New England Journal of Medicine* 372, no. 23 (June 4, 2015): 2235–42, doi:10.1056/NEJMsr1406261, Epub May 27, 2015.

15. H. L. Rehm et al., "ClinGen—the Clinical Genome Resource."

16. Christopher Weaver and Jeanne Whalen, "How Fake Cancer Drugs Entered U.S.," *Wall Street Journal*, July 20, 2012, www.wsj.com/articles/SB10001424052702303879604577410430607090226, accessed August 5, 2015.

17. I. Martincorena et al., "Tumor Evolution: High Burden and Pervasive Positive Selection of Somatic Mutations in Normal Human Skin," *Science* 348, no. 6237 (May 22, 2015): 880–86, doi:10.1126/science.aaa6806.

Chapter 1: The Century of Biology

1. R. J. Blendon, J. M. Benson, and J. O. Hero, "Public Trust in Physicians— U.S. Medicine in International Perspective," *New England Journal of Medicine* 371, no. 17 (October 23, 2014): 1570–72, doi:10.1056/ NEJMp1407373.
2. J. E. Oliver and T. Wood, "Medical Conspiracy Theories and Health Behaviors in the United States," *JAMA Internal Medicine* 174, no. 5 (May 2014): 817–18, doi:10.1001/jamainternmed.2014.190.
3. Associated Press, "How to Live Longer? Slow Eating!," *Daytona Beach* (FL) *Morning Journal*, August 10, 1960, 1, http://news.google.com/news papers?nid=1873&dat=19600809&id=IooeAAAAIBAJ&sjid=gcwEAA AAIBAJ&pg=6452,1440754, accessed August 6, 2015.
4. E. S. Lander, "Brave New Genome," *New England Journal of Medicine* 373, no. 1 (July 2, 2015): 5–8, doi:10.1056/NEJMp1506446, Epub June 3, 2015.
5. David Cyranoski and Sara Reardon, "Chinese Scientists Genetically Modify Human Embryos," *Nature* News, April 22, 2015.
6. Z. S. Morris, S. Wooding, and J. Grant, "The Answer Is 17 Years, What Is the Question: Understanding Time Lags in Translational Research," *Journal of the Royal Society of Medicine* 104, no. 12 (December 2011): 510–20, doi:10.1258/jrsm.2011.110180.
7. The photo of Dr. Coley is taken from https://en.wikipedia.org/wiki /William_Coley#mediaviewer/File:William_Coley_1892.jpg.
8. E. F. McCarthy, "The Toxins of William B. Coley and the Treatment of Bone and Soft-Tissue Sarcomas," *Iowa Orthopaedic Journal* 26 (2006): 154–58.
9. For more information about the Duke trials using the polio virus, go to the Preston Robert Tisch Brain Tumor Center of Duke University Medical Center, www.cancer.duke.edu/btc/modules/Research3/index .php?id=41.
10. D. T. Le et al., "PD-1 Blockade in Tumors with Mismatch-Repair Deficiency," *New England Journal of Medicine* 372, no. 26 (June 25, 2015): 2509–20, doi:10.1056/NEJMoa1500596, Epub May 30, 2015.
11. P. J. Parekh, L. A. Balart, and D. A. Johnson, "The Influence of the Gut Microbiome on Obesity, Metabolic Syndrome and Gastrointestinal Disease," *Clinical Translational Gastroenterology* 6 (June 18, 2015): E91, doi:10.1038/ctg.2015.16.

12. S. Gordon, "Élie Metchnikoff: Father of Natural Immunity," *European Journal of Immunology* 38, no. 12 (December 2008): 3257–64, doi:10.1002/eji.200838855, http://onlinelibrary.wiley.com/doi/10.1002/eji.200838855/pdf, accessed August 6, 2015.

Chapter 2: This Isn't Science Fiction

1. J. Quoidbach, D. T. Gilbert, and T. D. Wilson, "The End of History Illusion," *Science* 339, no. 6115 (January 4, 2013): 96–98, doi:10.1126/science.1229294.
2. Ibid.
3. J. Kirstein et al., "Proteotoxic Stress and Ageing Triggers the Loss of Redox Homeostasis Cross Cellular Compartments," *EMBO Journal* (July 29, 2015), pii: e201591711 (Epub ahead of print).
4. J. Labbadia and R. I. Morimoto, "Repression of the Heat Shock Response Is a Programmed Event at the Onset of Reproduction," *Molecular Cell* (July 22, 2015), pii: S1097–2765(15)00499–2, doi:10.1016/j.molcel.2015.06.027 (Epub ahead of print).
5. O. R. Jones et al., "Diversity of Ageing Across the Tree of Life," *Nature* 505, no. 7482 (January 9, 2014): 169–73, doi:10.1038/nature12789, Epub December 8, 2013. Also see "Surprising Diversity in Aging Revealed in Nature," Phys.org, December 8, 2013, http://phys.org/news/2013-12-diversity-aging-revealed-nature.html?.
6. D. W. Belsky et al., "Quantification of Biological Aging in Young Adults," *Proceedings of the National Academy of Sciences of the United States of America* 112, no. 30 (July 28, 2015): E4104–10, doi:10.1073/pnas.1506264112, Epub July 6, 2015.
7. Ariana Eunjung Cha, "Study of 1,000 38-Year-Olds Shows 'Biological Age' Ranges from 30 to 60," *Washington Post*, July 7, 2015, www.washingtonpost.com/news/to-your-health/wp/2015/07/07/study-of-1000-38-year-olds-shows-biological-age-ranges-from-30-to-60/?.
8. Belsky et al., "Quantification of Biological Aging in Young Adults."
9. For more about the heart age calculator, go to www.cdc.gov/vitalsigns/cardiovasculardisease/heartage.html.
10. For more information about Foundation Medicine's services, go to www.foundationmedicine.com.
11. Some have called immunotherapy the "fifth pillar" of cancer treatment after surgery, chemo, radiation, and drugs such as Gleevec and Herceptin that target cancer cells' mutations.
12. L. M. Abegglen et al., "Potential Mechanisms for Cancer Resistance in Elephants and Comparative Cellular Response to DNA Damage in Humans," *JAMA*. Published online October 08, 2015. doi:10.1001/jama

.2015.13134. Also see: Michael Sulak et al., "TP53 Copy Number Expansion Correlates with the Evolution of Increased Body Size and an Enhanced DNA Damage Response in Elephants," Cold Springs Harbor Laboratory, bioRxiv, a prepublication posting, October 6, 2015, http:// biorxiv.org/content/early/2015/10/06/028522.

13. D. P. Lane, "Cancer. p53, Guardian of the Genome," Nature 358, no. 6381 (July 2, 1992): 15–6.

14. For a wonderful chronicle of Massagué Solé's life and work, see Elizabeth Devita-Raeburn, "The Unintentional Scientist: Joan Massagué Was Having Too Much Fun to Notice He Was Building a Career—and Solving Problems of Cell Signaling and Cancer Metastasis," Howard Hughes Medical Institute Bulletin, August 2008, https://web.archive.org /web/20120905041353/http://www.hhmi.org/bulletin/aug2008/pdf /Scientist.pdf, accessed August 7, 2015.

15. J. L. Watkins et al., "Clinical Impact of Selective and Nonselective Beta-Blockers on Survival in Patients with Ovarian Cancer," Cancer (August 24, 2015), doi: 10.1002/cncr.29392. Epub ahead of print.

16. B. Dulken and A. Brunet, "Stem Cell Aging and Sex: Are We Missing Something?" Cell Stem Cell 16, no. 6 (June 4, 2015): 588–90, doi:10.1016/j.stem.2015.05.006.

17. C. Zhang et al., "Genetic Determinants of Telomere Length and Risk of Common Cancers: A Mendelian Randomization Study," Human Molecular Genetics 24, no. 18 (September 15, 2015): 5356-66, doi: 10.1093/ hmg/ddv252. Epub 2015 Jul 2.

18. "Antimicrobial Resistance: Tackling a Crisis for the Health and Wealth of Nations," Review on Antimicrobial Resistance, chaired by Jim O'Neill, December 2014, http://amr-review.org/sites/default/files/AMR%20Review% 20Paper%20-%20Tackling%20a%20crisis%20for%20the%20health %20and%20wealth%20of%20nations_1.pdf, accessed August 7, 2015.

19. Kirandeep Bhullar et al., "Antibiotic Resistance Is Prevalent in an Isolated Cave Microbiome," PLOS ONE 7, no. 4 (2012): E34953, doi:10.1371/ journal.pone.0034953.

20. L. L. Ling et al., "A New Antibiotic Kills Pathogens Without Detectable Resistance," Nature 517, no. 7535 (January 22, 2015): 455–59, doi:10.1038/nature14098, Epub January 7, 2015.

Chapter 3: The Future You

1. G. J. Xu et al., "Viral Immunology. Comprehensive Serological Profiling of Human Populations Using a Synthetic Human Virome," Science 348, no. 6239 (June 5, 2015): aaa0698, doi:10.1126/science.aaa0698. Also see Denise Grady, "New Test Traces a Person's Virus History," Boston Globe,

June 5, 2015, www.bostonglobe.com/business/2015/06/04/single-test -for-all-virus-exposure-opens-doors-for-researchers/uZ7DwhaIHXha1 ux1dtdb4K/story.html?.

2. J. Suez et al., "Artificial Sweeteners Induce Glucose Intolerance by Altering the Gut Microbiota," *Nature* 514, no. 7521 (October 9, 2014): 181–86, doi:10.1038/nature13793, Epub September 17, 2014.

3. N. H. Shah et al., "Proton Pump Inhibitor Usage and the Risk of Myocardial Infarction in the General Population," *PLOS ONE* 10, no. 6 (June 10, 2015): E0124653, doi:10.1371/journal.pone.0124653, eCollection 2015. Also see Kristin Magaldi, "Common OTC Antacids Increase Risk of Heart Attack up to 21%," *Medical Daily*, June 10, 2015, www.medicaldaily.com /common-otc-antacids-increase-risk-heart-attack-21-337594?.

4. Y. T. Ghebremariam et al., "Unexpected Effect of Proton Pump Inhibitors: Elevation of the Cardiovascular Risk Factor Asymmetric Dimethylarginine," *Circulation* 128, no. 8 (August 20, 2013): 845–53, doi:10.1161/ CIRCULATIONAHA.113.003602, Epub July 3, 2013.

5. Dominic Basulto, "How IBM Watson Will Impact Our Fight Against Cancer," *Washington Post*, May 6, 2015.

6. "Behind the Bloodshed: The Untold Story of America's Mass Killings," *USA Today*, www.gannett-cdn.com/GDContent/mass-killings/index .html#frequency, accessed August 7, 2015. Also see www.usatoday.com /story/news/nation/2013/09/16/mass-killings-data-map/2820423, accessed August 7, 2015.

7. C. Dufouil et al., "Older Age at Retirement Is Associated with Decreased Risk of Dementia," *European Journal of Epidemiology* 29, no. 5 (May 2014): 353–61, doi:10.1007/s10654-014-9906-3, Epub May 4, 2014.

8. A. L. Hansell et al., "Aircraft Noise and Cardiovascular Disease Near Heathrow Airport in London: Small Area Study," *British Medical Journal* 34 (October 8, 2013): F5432, doi:10.1136/bmj.f5432.

9. A. W. Correia et al., "Residential Exposure to Aircraft Noise and Hospital Admissions for Cardiovascular Diseases: Multi-Airport Retrospective Study," *British Medical Journal* 347 (October 8, 2013): F5561, doi:10.1136/bmj.f5561.

10. Gina Kolata, "Antibiotics Are Effective in Appendicitis, Study Says," *New York Times*, June 17, 2015, A17. Also see P. Salminen et al., "Antibiotic Therapy Vs. Appendectomy for Treatment of Uncomplicated Acute Appendicitis: The APPAC Randomized Clinical Trial," *Journal of the American Medical Association* 313, no. 23 (June 16, 2015): 2340–48, doi:10.1001/jama.2015.6154.

11. Q. Ke et al., "Defining and Identifying Sleeping Beauties in Science," *Proceedings of the National Academy of Sciences of the United States of America* 112, no. 24 (June 16, 2015): 7426–31, doi:10.1073/pnas.1424329112, Epub May 26, 2015.

12. A big thanks goes out to Jay Walker for letting me reprint these images of the Bills of Mortality from his private collection and library. To see a virtual tour of his library, go to www.walkerdigital.com/the-walker-library _video-tour.html.

13. Declan Butler, "When Google Got Flu Wrong," *Nature* News, February 13, 2013. Also see "Google Flu Trends Gets It Wrong Three Years Running," *Daily News* by *New Scientist*, March 13, 2014. Also see D. Lazer et al., "Big Data. The Parable of Google Flu: Traps in Big Data Analysis," *Science* 343, no. 6176 (March 14, 2014): 1203–5, doi:10.1126/science.1248506.

Chapter 4: The Dawn of Precision Medicine

1. Nicholas Wade, "Scientists Seek Ban on Method of Editing the Human Genome," *New York Times*, March 19, 2015.

2. D. Baltimore et al., "Biotechnology. A Prudent Path Forward for Genomic Engineering and Germline Gene Modification," *Science* 348, no. 6230 (April 3, 2015): 36–38, doi:10.1126/science.aab1028, Epub March 19, 2015.

3. Sharon Bernardi's story has been well reported by the media, especially in Europe. You can view a video of her pleas for change in preventing mitochondrial disease on YouTube, https://www.youtube.com /watch?v=Zb6NWmFLiDs.

4. For more about mitochondrial diseases, visit the Cleveland Clinic's website devoted to this area: https://my.clevelandclinic.org/health/diseases _conditions/hic-what-are-mitochondrial-diseases/hic_Myths_and_Facts _About_Mitochondrial_Diseases.

5. The "three-parent" technology for eliminating mitochondrial disorders is well described in a thorough piece by Ewen Callaway, "Reproductive Medicine: The Power of Three," *Nature*, News Feature, May 21, 2014.

6. R. Rubin, "Precision Medicine: The Future or Simply Politics?," *Journal of the American Medical Association* 17, no. 313 (March 17, 2015): 1089–91, doi:10.1001/jama.2015.0957.

7. B. Diouf et al., "Association of an Inherited Genetic Variant with Vincristine-Related Peripheral Neuropathy in Children with Acute Lymphoblastic Leukemia," *Journal of the American Medical Association* 313, no. 8 (February 24, 2015): 815–23, doi:10.1001/jama.2015.0894.

8. R. Rubin, "Precision Medicine: The Future or Simply Politics?"

9. For information about the Human Microbiome Project, go to National Institutes of Health's dedicated site for the project: http://hmpdacc.org.

10. Multiple studies now show the relationship between gut health and mental wellness. For a general overview, see the following: E. A. Mayer, K. Tillisch, and A. Gupta, "Gut/Brain Axis and the Microbiota," *Journal of Clinical Investigation* 125, no. 3 (March 2, 2015): 926–38, doi:10.1172/

JCI76304, Epub February 17, 2015. Also see C. Schmidt, "Mental Health: Thinking from the Gut," *Nature* 518, no. 7540 (February 26, 2015): S12–15, doi:10.1038/518S13a.

11. B. Chassaing, "Dietary Emulsifiers Impact the Mouse Gut Microbiota Promoting Colitis and Metabolic Syndrome," *Nature* 519, no. 7541 (March 5, 2015): 92–96, doi:10.1038/nature14232, Epub February 25, 2015.

12. Multiple studies now demonstrate an association between the state of the gut microbiome and depression. Here's one: G. De Palma et al., "Microbiota and Host Determinants of Behavioural Phenotype in Maternally Separated Mice," *Nature Communications* 6 (July 28, 2015): 7735, doi:10.1038/ncomms8735.

13. Anna Azvolinsky, "Gut Microbes Influence Circadian Clock," *Scientist*, April 16, 2014.

14. S. DeWeerdt, "Microbiome: A Complicated Relationship Status," *Nature* 508, no. 7496 (April 17, 2014): S61–63, doi:10.1038/508S61a. See, in particular, box 1, "Lean Operation: Does the Microbiota Determine the Success of Gastric Surgery?"

15. These remarks were made in the reporting of the study by the University of North Carolina at Charlotte: University of North Carolina at Charlotte, Office of Public Relations, "Study Links E. Coli Variety to Colorectal Cancer," news release, August 17, 2012, http://publicrelations.uncc.edu /news-events/news-releases/study-links-e-coli-variety-colorectal-cancer . The following is the study's official citation: Janelle C. Arthur et al., "Intestinal Inflammation Targets Cancer-Inducing Activity of the Microbiota," *Science* 338, no. 6103 (October 5, 2012), 120–23, doi:10.1126/ science.1224820, Epub August 16, 2012.

16. X. C. Dopico et al., "Widespread Seasonal Gene Expression Reveals Annual Differences in Human Immunity and Physiology," *Nature Communications* 6 (May 12, 2015): 7000, doi:10.1038/ncomms8000.

Chapter 5: Take the Two-Week Challenge

1. R. Katz, "Biomarkers and Surrogate Markers: An FDA Perspective," *NeuroRx* 1, no. 2 (April 2004): 189–95.

2. M. E. Tinetti, T. R. Fried, and C. M. Boyd, "Designing Health Care for the Most Common Chronic Condition—Multimorbidity," *Journal of the American Medical Association* 307, no. 23 (June 20, 2012): 2493–94, doi:10.1001/jama.2012.5265.

3. M. Rahman and A. B. Berenson, "Self-Perception of Weight and Its Association with Weight-Related Behaviors in Young, Reproductive-Aged

Women," *Obstetrics & Gynecology* 116, no. 6 (December 2010): 1274–80, doi:10.1097/AOG.0b013e3181fdfc47.

4. Benjamin Radford, "Forty Percent of Overweight Women Don't Know It," Discovery News, December 10, 2010, http://news.discovery.com /human/psychology/40-of-overweight-women-dont-know-it-101210 .htm, accessed August 7, 2015.

5. A. Lundahl, K. M. Kidwell, and T. D. Nelson, "Parental Underestimates of Child Weight: A Meta-analysis," *Pediatrics* 133, no. 3 (March 2014): E689–703, doi:10.1542/peds.2013-2690, Epub February 2, 2014. See also H. Y. Chen et al., "Personal and Parental Weight Misperception and Self-Reported Attempted Weight Loss in US Children and Adolescents, National Health and Nutrition Examination Survey, 2007–2008 and 2009–2010," *Preventing Chronic Disease* 11 (July 31, 2014): E132, doi:10.5888/pcd11.140123. Also see Benjamin Radford's coverage for *Discovery News*: "Most Americans Are Overweight But Don't Know It," June 17, 2014.

6. Katherine Hobson, "Many Kids Who Are Obese or Overweight Don't Know It," NPR Health, July 23, 2014, www.npr.org: http://www.npr .org/sections/health-shots/2014/07/23/334091461/many-kids-who -are-obese-and-overweight-dont-know-it.

7. G. G. Kuhnle et al., "Association Between Sucrose Intake and Risk of Overweight and Obesity in a Prospective Sub-Cohort of the European Prospective Investigation into Cancer in Norfolk (EPIC-Norfolk)," *Public Health Nutrition* (February 23, 2015): 1–10 (Epub ahead of print).

8. S. Gill et al., "Time-Restricted Feeding Attenuates Age-Related Cardiac Decline in Drosophila," *Science* 347, no. 6227 (March 13, 2015): 1265–69, doi:10.1126/science.1256682. Also see Michael Price, "You Are When You Eat," San Diego State University News Center, March 12, 2015, http://universe.sdsu.edu/sdsu_newscenter/news_story .aspx?sid=75480.

9. Ellie Zolfagharifard, "400,000-Year-Old Teeth Reveal First Evidence of Man-Made Pollution—and Show the 'Caveman Diet' Really Was Balanced," DailyMail.com (UK), June 17, 2015, www.dailymail.co.uk /sciencetech/article-3128818/400-000-year-old-teeth-reveal-evidence -man-pollution-shows-caveman-diet-really-balanced.html, accessed August 8, 2015.

10. A. Pan et al., "Red Meat Consumption and Mortality: Results from 2 Prospective Cohort Studies," *Archives of Internal Medicine* 172, no. 7 (April 9, 2012): 555–63, doi:10.1001/archinternmed.2011.2287, Epub March 12, 2012.

11. M. Nagao et al., "Meat Consumption in Relation to Mortality from Cardiovascular Disease Among Japanese Men and Women," *European*

Journal of Clinical Nutrition 66, no. 6 (June 2012): 687–93. doi:10.1038/ejcn.2012.6, Epub February 15, 2012.

12. R. Micha, S. K. Wallace, and D. Mozaffarian, "Red and Processed Meat Consumption and Risk of Incident Coronary Heart Disease, Stroke, and Diabetes Mellitus: A Systematic Review and Meta-analysis," *Circulation* 121, no. 21 (June 1, 2010): 2271–83, doi:10.1161/CIRCULATION AHA.109.924977, Epub May 17, 2010.

13. The debate about the risk factors related to the consumption of red meat was well explained by Patrick J. Skerrett, "Study Urges Moderation in Red Meat Intake," *Harvard Health* (blog), March 13, 2012, www.health.harvard.edu/blog/study-urges-moderation-in-red-meat-intake-201203134490.

14. "Nearly 7 in 10 Americans Take Prescription Drugs, Mayo Clinic, Olmsted Medical Center Find," Mayo Clinic News Network, June 19, 2013, http://newsnetwork.mayoclinic.org.

15. Sumathi Reddy, "Why Seven Hours of Sleep Might Be Better Than Eight," *Wall Street Journal*, July 21, 2014, www.wsj.com/articles/sleep-experts -close-in-on-the-optimal-nights-sleep-1405984970?mod=trending_ now_1.

Chapter 6: The Danger of Misinformation

1. R. T. Hasty et al., "Wikipedia Vs. Peer-Reviewed Medical Literature for Information About the 10 Most Costly Medical Conditions," *Journal of the American Osteopathic Association,* 114, no. 5 (May 2014): 368–73, doi:10.7556/jaoa.2014.035.

2. B. Nyhan and J. Reifler, "Does Correcting Myths About the Flu Vaccine Work? An Experimental Evaluation of the Effects of Corrective Information," *Vaccine* 33, no. 3 (January 9, 2015): 459–64, doi:10.1016/j.vaccine .2014.11.017, Epub December 8, 2014.

3. Dan Kahan, "What Is Motivated Reasoning and How Does It Work?," *Science + Religion Today* (blog), May 4, 2011, www.scienceandreligion-today.com/2011/05/04/what-is-motivated-reasoning-and-how-does -it-work.

4. Building on the observation that milkmaids were generally immune to smallpox, Jenner scraped the pus from cowpox blisters on the hand of a milkmaid patient of his named Sarah Neimes (who caught cowpox from a Gloucester cow named Blossom). On May 14, 1796, he then injected it into an eight-year-old boy who was the son of Jenner's gardener, named James Phipps. The boy was later injected with smallpox-containing material twice, and nothing happened. By the way, *vacca* means "cow" in Latin; hence the name *vaccine*.

5. To read about the government's updated dietary guidelines, go to www .health.gov. Specifically, go to www.health.gov/dietaryguidelines/2015 -scientific-report/06-chapter-1/d1-2.asp.

6. J. R. Biesiekierski et al., "Gluten Causes Gastrointestinal Symptoms in Subjects Without Celiac Disease: A Double-Blind Randomized Placebo-Controlled Trial," *American Journal of Gastroenterology* 106, no. 3 (March 2011): 508–14, quiz 515, doi:10.1038/ajg.2010.487, Epub January 11, 2011.

7. J. R. Biesiekierski et al., "No Effects of Gluten in Patients with Self-Reported Non Celiac Gluten Sensitivity After Dietary Reduction of Fermentable, Poorly Absorbed, Short-Chain Carbohydrates," *Gastro-enterology* 145, no. 2 (August 2013): 320–28.e1-3, doi:10.1053/j.gastro .2013.04.051, Epub May 4, 2013.

8. Ross Pomeroy, "Non-Celiac Gluten Sensitivity May Not Exist," Real ClearScience.com, May 15, 2014.

9. "Davos 2015—Let Food Be Thy Medicine," YouTube video, 46:10, published on January 24, 2015, by the World Economic Forum (http://www .weforum.org), https://youtu.be/f26wfQBf1s.

10. D. Ornish et al., "Intensive Lifestyle Changes May Affect the Progression of Prostate Cancer," *Journal of Urology*, 174, no. 3 (September 2005): 1065–69; discussion 1069–70.

11. A. R. Kristal et al., "Baseline Selenium Status and Effects of Selenium and Vitamin E Supplementation on Prostate Cancer Risk," *Journal of the National Cancer Institute* 106, no. 3 (March 2014): djt456, doi:10.1093/ jnci/djt456, Epub February 22, 2014.

12. Johns Hopkins Medicine, "Bad Luck of Random Mutations Plays Predominant Role in Cancer, Study Shows—Statistical Modeling Links Cancer Risk with Number of Stem Cell Divisions," news release, January 1, 2015, www.hopkinsmedicine.org/news/media/releases/bad_luck_of_random _mutations_plays_predominant_role_in_cancer_study_shows.

13. C. Tomasetti and B. Vogelstein, "Cancer Etiology. Variation in Cancer Risk Among Tissues Can Be Explained by the Number of Stem Cell Divisions," *Science* 347, no. 6217 (January 2, 2015): 78–81, doi:10.1126/ science.1260825.

14. This quote by Tomasetti and Vogelstein was articulated in the addendum to the news release added January 7, 2015: http://www.hopkinsmedicine .org/news/media/releases/bad_luck_of_random_mutations_plays_pre dominant_role_in_cancer_study_shows.

15. Seth Rakoff-Nahoum, "Why Cancer and Inflammation?," *Yale Journal of Biological Medicine* 79 (December 2006): 123–30.

16. R. B. Haynes, "BMJUpdates+, A New *Free* Service for Evidence-Based Clinical Practice," *Evidence Based Nursing* 8, no. 2 (April 2005): 39, doi:10.1136/ebn.8.2.39.

17. Richard Horton, "Offline: What Is Medicine's 5 Sigma?" *Lancet* 385 (April 2015).

18. For an engaging read about hype in medical news, see Julia Belluz, "This Is Why You Shouldn't Believe That Exciting New Medical Study," Vox, last modified August 5, 2015, www.vox.com/2015/3/23/8264355/research -study-hype.

19. J. D. Schoenfeld and J. P. Ioannidis, "Is Everything We Eat Associated with Cancer? A Systematic Cookbook Review," *American Journal of Clinical Nutrition* 97, no. 1 (January 2013): 127–34, doi:10.3945/ajcn.112.047142, Epub November 28, 2012.

20. J. P. Ioannidis, "Why Most Published Research Findings Are False," *PLOS Medicine* 2, no. 8 (August 2005): E124, Epub August 30, 2005.

21. H. Bastian, "Seventy-five Trials and Eleven Systematic Reviews a Day: How Will We Ever Keep Up?" *PLOS Medicine* 7, no. 9 (September 21, 2010): E1000326, doi:10.1371/journal.pmed.1000326.

22. Jeffrey Beall, "List of Predatory Publishers," Scholarly Open Access blog, last modified January 2, 2014, http://scholarlyoa.com/2014/01/02/list -of-predatory-publishers-2014/.

23. P. Autier, "Vitamin D Status and Ill Health: A Systematic Review," *Lancet Diabetes Endocrinology* 2, no. 1 (January 2014): 76–89, doi:10.1016/ S2213-8587(13)70165-7, Epub December 6, 2013.

24. I. R. Reid, "Effects of Vitamin D Supplements on Bone Mineral Density: A Systematic Review and Meta-Analysis," *Lancet* 383, no. 9912 (January 11, 2014): 146–55, doi:10.1016/S0140-6736(13)61647-5, Epub October 11, 2013.

25. E. S. LeBlanc et al., "Screening for Vitamin D Deficiency: Systematic Review for the U.S. Preventive Services Task Force," *Annals of Internal Medicine* 162, no. 2 (January 20, 2015): 109–22, doi:10.7326/M14-1659.

26. Anahad O'Conner, "Fish Oil Claims Not Well Supported," *New York Times*, March 30, 2015, http://well.blogs.nytimes.com/2015/03/30/fish -oil-claims-not-supported-by-research.

27. For a quick summary of some of these studies and their controversy, see Melinda Wenner Moyer, "Fish Oil Supplement Research Remains Murky," *Scientific American*, September 24, 2012. Also see Howard LeWine, "Fish Oil: Friend or Foe?," *Harvard Health Blog*, July 12, 2013, www.health .harvard.edu/blog/fish-oil-friend-or-foe-201307126467.

28. R. Marchioli, "Early Protection Against Sudden Death by N-3 Polyunsaturated Fatty Acids After Myocardial Infarction: Time-Course Analysis of the Results of the Gruppo Italiano per lo Studio della Sopravvivenza nell'Infarto Miocardico (GISSI)-Prevenzione," *Circulation* 105, no. 16 (April 23, 2002): 1897–903.

29. Risk and Prevention Study Collaborative Group, M.C. Roncaglioni et al., "N-3 Fatty Acids in Patients with Multiple Cardiovascular Risk Factors,"

New England Journal of Medicine 368, no. 19 (May 9, 2013): 1800–1808, doi:10.1056/NEJMoa1205409.

Chapter 7: A Body in Motion Tends to Stay Lucky

1. CDC Newsroom, "One in Five Adults Meet Overall Physical Activity Guidelines," news release, May 2, 2013, www.cdc.gov/media/releases /2013/p0502-physical-activity.html.
2. I. M. Lee et al., "Effect of Physical Inactivity on Major Non-communicable Diseases Worldwide: An Analysis of Burden of Disease and Life Expectancy," *Lancet* 380, no. 9838 (July 21, 2012): 219–29, doi:10.1016/ S0140-6736(12)61031-9.
3. J. G. van Uffelen et al., "Sitting-Time, Physical Activity, and Depressive Symptoms in Mid-Aged Women," *American Journal of Preventive Medicine* 45, no. 3 (September 2013): 276–81, doi:10.1016/j.amepre.2013 .04.009.
4. See the WHO's global recommendations on physical activity for health, www.who.int/dietphysicalactivity/factsheet_recommendations/en.
5. S. C. Moore et al., "Leisure Time Physical Activity of Moderate to Vigorous Intensity and Mortality: A Large Pooled Cohort Analysis," *PLOS Medicine* 9, no. 11 (2012): E1001335, doi:10.1371/journal.pmed.1001335, Epub November 6, 2012.
6. S. G. Lakoski, "Midlife Cardiorespiratory Fitness, Incident Cancer, and Survival After Cancer in Men: The Cooper Center Longitudinal Study," *JAMA Oncology* 1, no. 2 (May 1, 2015): 231–37, doi:10.1001/jamaoncol .2015.0226.
7. A. S. Betof et al., "Modulation of Murine Breast Tumor Vascularity, Hypoxia and Chemotherapeutic Response by Exercise," *Journal of the National Cancer Institute* 107, no. 5 (2015): djv040, doi:10.1093/jnci/djv040. Also see Duke Medicine, "Exercise Slows Tumor Growth, Improves Chemotherapy in Mouse Cancers," ScienceDaily, last modified March 16, 2015, www.sciencedaily.com/releases/2015/03/150316185446.htm.
8. Benjamin L. Willis et al., "Midlife Fitness and the Development of Chronic Conditions in Later Life," *Archives of Internal Medicine* 172, no. 17 (September 24, 2012): 1333–40, doi:10.1001/archinternmed.2012.3400.
9. L. L. Craft et al., "Evidence That Women Meeting Physical Activity Guidelines Do Not Sit Less: An Observational Inclinometry Study," *International Journal of Behavioral Nutrition and Physical Activity* 9 (October 4, 2012): 122, doi:10.1186/1479-5868-9-122.
10. R. R. Wolfe, "The Underappreciated Role of Muscle in Health and Disease," *American Journal of Clinical Nutrition* 84, no. 3 (September 2006): 475–82.

11. A. P. Wroblewski et al., "Chronic Exercise Preserves Lean Muscle Mass in Masters Athletes," *Physician and Sportsmedicine* 39, no. 3 (September 2011): 172–88, doi:10.3810/psm.2011.09.1933.
12. Gretchen Reynolds, "How Much Exercise Is Enough?," *New York Times*, April 15, 2015.
13. H. Arem et al., "Leisure Time Physical Activity and Mortality: A Detailed Pooled Analysis of the Dose-Response Relationship," *JAMA Internal Medicine* 175, no. 6 (June 2015): 959–67, doi:10.1001/jamaintern med.2015.0533.
14. K. Gebel et al., "Effect of Moderate to Vigorous Physical Activity on All-Cause Mortality in Middle-Aged and Older Australians," *JAMA Internal Medicine* 175, no. 6 (June 2015): 970–77, doi:10.1001/jamaintern med.2015.0541.
15. L. B. B. Brito et al., "Ability to Sit and Rise from the Floor as a Predictor of All-Cause Mortality," *European Journal of Preventive Cardiology* (2012), doi:10.1177/2047487312471759.

Chapter 8: Wonder Drugs That Work

1. Matt McCarthy, "Science of Nap Time," *Sports Illustrated*, April 13, 2015.
2. Ricardo S. Osorio et al., "Sleep-Disordered Breathing Advances Cognitive Decline in the Elderly," *Neurology* (April 2015), doi:10.1212/ WNL.0000000000001566.
3. W. C. Winter et al., "Measuring Circadian Advantage in Major League Baseball: A 10-Year Retrospective Study," *International Journal of Sports Physiology and Performance* 4, no. 3 (September 2009): 394–401.
4. For more about the National Sleep Foundation's recommendations and related studies, go to www.nationalsleepfoundation.org.
5. J. Zhang et al., "Extended Wakefulness: Compromised Metabolics in and Degeneration of Locus Ceruleus Neurons," *Journal of Neuroscience* 34, no. 12 (March 19, 2014): 4418–31, doi:10.1523/JNEUROSCI.5025-12.2014.
6. Alice Park, "The Power of Sleep," *Time*, September 22, 2014.
7. B. A. Plog et al., "Biomarkers of Traumatic Injury Are Transported from Brain to Blood via the Glymphatic System," *Journal of Neuroscience* 35, no. 2 (January 14, 2015): 518–26, doi:10.1523/JNEUROSCI.3742-14.2015.
8. A. Louveau et al., "Structural and Functional Features of Central Nervous System Lymphatic Vessels," *Nature* 523, no. 7560 (July 16, 2015): 337–41, doi:10.1038/nature14432, Epub June 1, 2015.
9. Park, "Power of Sleep."
10. Ibid.
11. Melinda Beck, "The Joy of Researching the Benefits of Sex," *Wall Street Journal*, May 3, 2011.

12. For a fantastic read of this history couched in modern science, see Maria Konnikova, "The Power of Touch," *New Yorker*, March 4, 2015. Also see William J. Cromie, "Of Hugs and Hormones," *Harvard University Gazette*, June 11, 1998, http://news.harvard.edu/gazette/1998/06.11/OfHugs andHormon.html.

13. M. Carlson and F. Earls, "Psychological and Neuroendocrinological Sequelae of Early Social Deprivation in Institutionalized Children in Romania," *Annals of the New York Academy of Sciences* 807 (January 15, 1997): 419–28.

14. To see a full bibliography of Tiffany Field's work with colleagues on the power of touch, go to https://www6.miami.edu/touch-research/Research .html.

15. S. Cohen et al., "Does Hugging Provide Stress-Buffering Social Support? A Study of Susceptibility to Upper Respiratory Infection and Illness," *Psychological Science* 26, no. 2 (February 2015): 135–47, doi:10.1177/0956797614559284, Epub December 19, 2014.

16. David J. Linden, *Touch: The Science of Hand, Heart, and Mind* (New York: Viking, 2015).

17. Some of the material in this section is adapted from an op-ed article I wrote, "The 2,000-Year-Old Wonder Drug," *New York Times*, December 11, 2012.

18. P. M. Rothwell et al., "Effect of Daily Aspirin on Long-Term Risk of Death Due to Cancer: Analysis of Individual Patient Data from Randomised Trials," *Lancet* 377, no. 9759 (January 1, 2011): 31–41, doi:10.1016/ S0140-6736(10)62110-1, Epub December 6, 2010.

19. P. M. Rothwell et al., "Effect of Daily Aspirin on Risk of Cancer Metastasis: A Study of Incident Cancers During Randomised Controlled Trials," *Lancet* 379, no. 9826 (April 28, 2012): 1591–601, doi:10.1016/S0140- 6736(12)60209-8, Epub March 21, 2012.

20. P. M. Rothwell et al., "Short-Term Effects of Daily Aspirin on Cancer Incidence, Mortality, and Non-Vascular Death: Analysis of the Time Course of Risks and Benefits in 51 Randomised Controlled Trials," *Lancet* 379, no. 9826 (April 28, 2012):1602–12, doi:10.1016/S0140- 6736(11)61720-0, Epub March 21, 2012.

21. Yin Cao, postdoctoral research fellow, Harvard School of Public Health, Boston; Eric Jacobs, PhD, strategic director, pharmacoepidemiology, American Cancer Society; April 19, 2015, presentation, American Association for Cancer Research meeting, Philadelphia.

22. S. F. Nielsen, B. G. Nordestgaard, and S. E. Bojesen, "Statin Use and Reduced Cancer-Related Mortality," *New England Journal of Medicine* 367, no. 19 (November 8, 2012): 1792–802, doi:10.1056/NEJMoa1201735. Also see S. F. Nielsen, B. G. Nordestgaard, and S. E. Bojesen, "Statin Use and Reduced Cancer-Related Mortality," *New England Journal of Medicine* 368, no. 6 (February 7, 2013): 576–77, doi:10.1056/NEJMc1214827.

23. C. R. Cardwell et al., "Statin Use and Survival from Lung Cancer: A Population-Based Cohort Study," *Cancer Epidemiology, Biomarkers & Prevention* 24, no. 5 (May 2015): 833–41, doi:10.1158/1055-9965.EPI-15-0052.

24. Leah Lawrence, "Statins Linked with Reduced Liver Cancer in Low-Rate Areas," Cancer Network, March 19, 2015, www.cancernetwork.com/gastrointestinal-cancer/statins-linked-reduced-liver-cancer-low-rate-areas#sthash.mYYAMgXP.dpuf.

25. L. C. Harshman, "Statin Use at the Time of Initiation of Androgen Deprivation Therapy and Time to Progression in Patients with Hormone-Sensitive Prostate Cancer," *JAMA Oncology* 1, no. 4 (July 1, 2015): 495–504, doi:10.1001/jamaoncol.2015.0829.

26. C. R. Cardwell et al., "Statin Use After Colorectal Cancer Diagnosis and Survival: A Population-Based Cohort Study," *Journal of Clinical Oncology* 32, no. 28 (October 1, 2014): 3177–83, doi:10.1200/JCO.2013.54.4569, Epub August 4, 2014.

27. T. J. Murtola et al., "Statin Use and Breast Cancer Survival: A Nationwide Cohort Study from Finland," *PLOS ONE* 9, no. 10 (October 20, 2014): E110231, doi:10.1371/journal.pone.0110231. eCollection 2014.

28. A. Pursnani et al., "Guideline-Based Statin Eligibility, Coronary Artery Calcification, and Cardiovascular Events," *Journal of the American Medical Association* 314, no. 2 (July 14, 2015): 134–41, doi:10.1001/jama.2015.7515.

29. J. M. Patel et al., "Randomized Double-Blind Placebo-Controlled Trial of 40 Mg/Day of Atorvastatin in Reducing the Severity of Sepsis in Ward Patients (ASEPSIS Trial)," *Critical Care* 16, no. 6 (December 11, 2012): R231, doi:10.1186/cc11895. For an intriguing commentary on this phenomenon, see David S. Fedson and Steven M. Opal, "Can Statins Help Treat Ebola?," *New York Times*, August 15, 2014.

Chapter 9: The Butterfly Effect

1. Malcolm Gladwell, *Blink: The Power of Thinking Without Thinking* (New York: Little, Brown, 2005).

2. Excerpt from Gladwell, *Blink: The Power of Thinking Without Thinking*, iBooks. https://itun.es/us/wByuv.

3. Michael Kimmelman, "ART; Absolutely Real? Absolutely Fake?," *New York Times*, August 4, 1991.

4. Charles Duhigg, *The Power of Habit: Why We Do What We Do in Life and Business* (New York: Random House, 2012).

5. For a comprehensive review of perceptual intuition, see Benedict Carey, "Brain Calisthenics for Abstract Ideas," *New York Times*, June 6, 2011. Also see Carey, "Learning to See Data," *New York Times*, March 27, 2015.

6. To learn more about Muhammad Yunus and his work, visit the Yunus
   Center's website at http://muhammadyunus.org.
7. To read Lorenz's original academic paper, go to http://eaps4.mit.edu
   /research/Lorenz/Butterfly_1972.pdf.
8. J. Lightwood and S. A. Glantz, "The Effect of the California Tobacco
   Control Program on Smoking Prevalence, Cigarette Consumption, and
   Healthcare Costs: 1989–2008," *PLOS ONE* 8, no. 2 (2013): E47145,
   doi:10.1371/journal.pone.0047145, Epub February 13, 2013.
9. Federal Trade Commission. Federal Trade Commission Cigarette Report
   for 2012.
10. "Youth and Tobacco Use," Centers for Disease Control and Preven-
    tion, last modified July 24, 2015, www.cdc.gov/tobacco/data_statistics
    /fact_sheets/youth_data/tobacco_use/index.htm.
11. Aldous Huxley, *Brave New World* (New York: Random House, 1932),
    chap. 17.

Index

About the Author

Dr. David B. Agus is a professor of medicine and engineering at the University of Southern California Keck School of Medicine and Viterbi School of Engineering and heads USC's Westside Cancer Center and the Center for Applied Molecular Medicine. He is one of the world's leading cancer doctors and the cofounder of two pioneering personalized medicine companies, Navigenics and Applied Proteomics. Dr. Agus is an international leader in new technologies and approaches for personalized health care and a contributor to CBS News. His first two books, *The End of Illness* and *A Short Guide to a Long Life*, were both *New York Times* and international bestsellers, with *The End of Illness* hitting number one on the list.

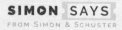